NATURAL HIGHS

FOR BODY AND SOUL

REMEDIES, RITUALS AND TECHNIQUES
TO BANISH EVERYDAY ENERGY LOWS

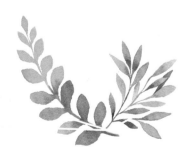

An Hachette UK Company
www.hachette.co.uk

First published in Great Britain in 2005 by Hamlyn,
an imprint of Octopus Publishing Group Ltd
Carmelite House, 50 Victoria Embankment,
London EC4Y 0DZ
www.octopusbooks.co.uk

This edition published in 2019 by Pyramid,
an imprint of Octopus Publishing Group Ltd

ISBN 978-0-75373-392-9

A CIP catalogue record for this book is available
from the British Library

Printed and bound in China

For the Pyramid edition:
Publisher: Lucy Pessell
Designer: Hannah Coughlin
Production Manager: Grace O'Byrne

10 9 8 7 6 5 4 3 2 1

Disclaimer
The information and advice contained in this book
are intended as a general guide. This book is not
intended to replace treatment by a qualified
practitioner. Neither the author nor the publishers
can be held responsible for claims arising from the
inappropriate use of any remedy.

Yoga
(see pages 50–51 and 124–125)
These postures can be practised quite safely; but
to enjoy the full benefits of yoga, it is advisable
to go to a yoga class with a trained teacher. If
you are pregnant, are unfit or have a medical
problem, consult your doctor before performing
the postures.

Acupressure and reflexology
(see pages 52–53, 64–65, 68–69 and 102–103)
Do not practise these routines if you have a heart
condition, phlebitis, breast or lymphatic cancer,
or in the first 16 weeks of pregnancy. Also do
not use if your hands or feet have an infectious
skin condition, are bruised or cut. If you have any
other condition you are concerned about, such as
diabetes, check with your doctor before treating
yourself.

Chi kung
(see pages 78–79)
These poses are quite safe to practise, but to learn
chi kung fully it is advisable to attend a class. If you
have a health problem, consult your doctor before
practising chi kung.

CONTENTS

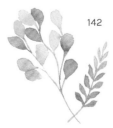

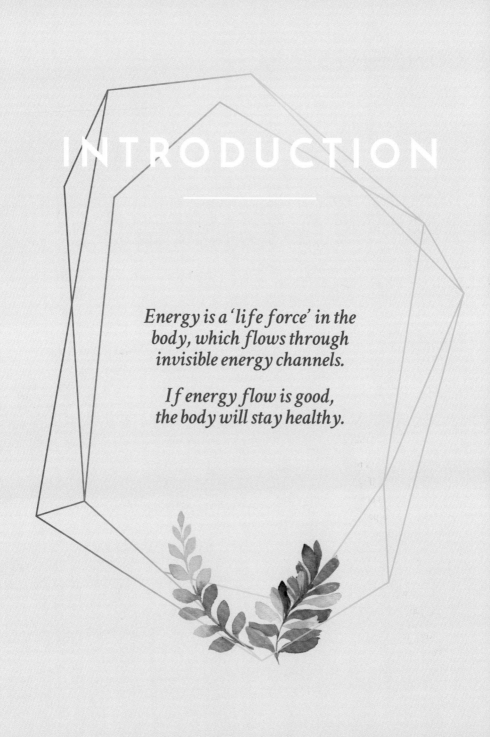

INTRODUCTION

Energy is a 'life force' in the body, which flows through invisible energy channels.

If energy flow is good, the body will stay healthy.

In our lives today we often complain about a lack of energy. Our lives have become overcomplicated; we try to do too much, running ourselves ragged and ending up feeling tired and exhausted. Many of us are forced to work long hours, often while looking after a family as well, and there is precious little time left for us. Pollutants in the environment, daily commuting, a poor diet and a lack of sleep and exercise all take their toll on our energy levels. Added to this, as we get older our energy levels naturally decline, which makes it even more important to stay healthy and maintain energy throughout life.

When we look at energy levels from the Western perspective, they are intrinsically linked to the life we lead. We obtain our energy from the food we eat, and the energetic ups and downs we suffer are caused by fluctuating blood-sugar levels if meals are missed or eaten late, or if we regularly ingest toxins by smoking or drinking alcohol, for example.

The Eastern view of energy is quite different: energy is seen from a holistic point of view, looking at the health of the mind, body and spirit of an individual. Eastern philosophers believe that they all need to be in balance for true wellbeing. Energy is a 'life force' in the body, which flows through invisible energy channels. When an Eastern health diagnosis is made, the energy flow is studied in detail and any blockage or stagnancy is treated. Overall, however, the philosophy is preventative, with the belief that if the energy flow is good, the body will stay healthy.

This book aims to show you how to keep your energy levels balanced holistically, because even if your diet and general lifestyle are good, you can be drained daily by stress, upsets at work or problems with friends and family. The Instant Energizers section (see pages 36–141) contains over 70 'mini' exercises or therapies to suit different times of the day. Each 'energizer' takes only a matter of minutes, so you can do it when you feel your energy levels dropping.

In time, you will discover how to listen to your all your body's energy needs and know when the time is right for an empowering mantra, a stimulating herbal tea or a relaxing neck and shoulder massage exercise to get you through another busy day.

Keeping your mind, body and spirit healthy will change your life, as you take time out to become more in tune with yourself and at peace with the world.

In the West today we seem to be working harder than ever with many people complaining of low energy levels or feeling 'tired all the time'.

1

WHAT IS ENERGY?

THE WESTERN CONCEPT OF ENERGY

In the Western world we see energy as our drive or enthusiasm for achieving our objectives in day-to-day life. Our energy is obtained from food and energy levels are measured in calories (kilocalories or kilojoules). Our daily intake of food provides the energy needed for our muscles and organs to function well. Eating a healthy, balanced diet gives us the optimum energy levels we require.

But in the West today we seem to be working harder than ever with many people complaining of low energy levels or feeling 'tired all the time', which basically results from neglecting normal physical, dietary and emotional needs. In today's busy world, people often eat on the go, indulging in a quick energy fix of sugary or processed foods when they need a pick-me-up. They regularly take limited exercise (if at all), have little time to relax and deprive themselves of sleep – no wonder, then, that energy levels often remain low.

THE BENEFITS OF A GOOD DIET

Energy highs and lows relate to fluctuating blood-sugar levels – the more balanced and steady they are, the better we feel. Skipping meals or dieting disrupts these levels, lowering your energy. Blood-sugar levels start to drop within four hours of eating, so to counteract the inevitable dip eat three smaller meals (with some healthy snacks in between) at regular times throughout the day, rather than just eating two large meals a day.

Most of the energy from food comes in the form of carbohydrates (basically starches and sugars) and fats that 'fuel' the body. This food energy is released into the body with the help of micronutrients – vitamins and minerals that derive from the fruit and vegetables you eat. Protein provides some energy and keeps blood-sugar levels stable but it is mainly used for body maintenance and repair. Eating sugary or processed foods, which are often full of artificial additives, preservatives and flavourings, disrupts your energy levels. For example, if you snack on cakes or biscuits you get an instant burst of energy from the fast sugar release, but soon after your energy plummets again, leaving you tired and craving yet more sugar. Snacks such as fresh fruit and nuts, however, raise blood-sugar levels much more gradually, giving you a more sustained energy supply that keeps you going longer.

If you eat a healthy balanced diet but still complain of lethargy, it may be because you don't drink enough water. Being dehydrated can make you feel tired, so drink a glass of still water at room temperature every hour during the day, or keep a bottle of still mineral water by you. However, avoid drinking with meals as it hinders digestion.

THE RIGHT BALANCE OF FOOD

To keep you healthy and your energy levels stable, it is best to eat a varied and balanced diet with plenty of unrefined food and fresh produce, ideally organic. Include at least five portions of fruit and vegetables for essential vitamins and minerals; three or four portions of complex carbohydrates (unrefined) such as wholewheat bread, brown pasta and rice, potatoes and pulses; one or two portions of protein, such as fish (oily fish is ideal), meat, poultry, tofu, seeds or eggs plus a small amount of fat such as olive oil or butter.

HEALTHY SNACKS

Rebalance your blood-sugar levels throughout the day with these high-energy foods:

dried fruit and nuts (salt-free)

fresh fruit

seeds (sunflower or pumpkin)

raw vegetables with sour cream dip

cereal bars (sugar-free)

hummus and crispbread

low-fat yogurt

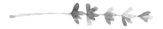

THE IMPORTANCE OF SLEEP

Sleep is vital for a healthy body and mind. It allows the body to rest and restore itself. While we sleep, the healing and repair of cells, tissues, bones, muscles, nerves and organs takes place. When we are deprived of sleep, even for one night, our coping strategies weaken and we find it difficult to function properly.

We feel fatigued and exhausted, lack concentration and have depleted energy levels. Worries and anxiety can cause disrupted sleep patterns, so any niggling issues need to be worked through before going to bed (see Late-night Cleansers, pages 126–141). While some people can manage on a few hours, an average of 7–8 hours' sleep a night is normally enough to refresh, revitalize and re-energize our bodies.

A REGULAR EXERCISE ROUTINE

Taking regular exercise tones your body muscles and improves how efficiently your organs work, particularly your heart and lungs. It makes you feel good about yourself, improves your sleep and boosts your overall energy so that you achieve more. You also benefit from the 'feel good factor' – the result of endorphins, the 'happy hormones' being released into the bloodstream.

The latest recommendation is for 30 minutes' exercise on most days of the week (you can even do it in 10-minute bouts if half an hour is hard to find). Ideally, combine some aerobic activity (where you work your lungs and heart hard until slightly breathless), such as fast walking, running, swimming or cycling, with stretching exercises to improve muscle suppleness; even some household chores, such as vacuuming, scrubbing floors or gardening, are aerobic activities. It is a good idea to also include some weight-bearing exercise such as tennis, dancing or skipping to strengthen your muscles and improve your bone density.

THE EASTERN CONCEPT OF ENERGY

Even when you have worked hard at balancing your energy levels by eating well, being more active, getting enough sleep and keeping your stress levels in check, you may still feel lethargic or listless and not really know why. According to the Eastern philosophy of energy you may be suffering from an energy blockage or stagnancy in one of your body's meridians (energy channels) that flow through your body or one of the chakras (spiritual energy centres). Eastern medicine aims to be preventative and works with the body's strengths and its natural inclination to heal itself. It looks at the body holistically and believes that either illness starts as an emotional upset or imbalance in one of the chakras that, if not dealt with, eventually manifests itself as a physical illness or illness in a part of the body that results from an emotional energy disturbance in energy points along one or more meridians.

CHI, PRANA OR KI

In traditional Chinese medicine the body's energy or life force is known as *chi* (*qi*). It is an invisible form of energy, similar to electromagnetic energy, that flows through a set of meridians or channels affecting the health of every cell in the body.

In Indian Ayurvedic medicine the body's energy force is known as *prana*. It moves through numerous meridians in the body, and needs to be balanced for good health in the same way as in traditional Chinese medicine. In Japanese medicine the energy flow is called *ki*, and it works with the same meridians as in the Chinese system.

THE MERIDIANS OR NADIS

Chi (*qi*) or the Japanese *ki* moves around the body through 12 main meridians and several minor ones. Six of the main meridians are yin and six are yang. Yin and yang are opposing forces that affect everything; one cannot act without the other: they are interdependent. Yin comes from the earth and is dark, passive and feminine, whereas yang comes from the sun and is light, active and male. To achieve optimum energy levels at all times, you need to keep a balance of both in the body.

Each main meridian connects to and is related to an organ or function. The yin meridians relate to the heart, liver, kidney, lung, pericardium (part of the heart) and spleen. The yang meridians relate to the triple-warmer (a metabolic zone), stomach, bladder, gall bladder, small intestines and large intestines. There are two extra meridians: the governor and conception. It is along these 14 meridians that 365 of the acupuncture points are found, all of which are named and numbered. When these are stimulated, stagnant or blocked energy can be shifted so that *chi* moves freely once again. When an imbalance is found in a person's body it can be related to an excessive emotional response such as rage, intense grief or sorrow or anxiety. For example, someone who suffers inappropriate anger can experience an imbalance in the liver. The Indian energy, *prana*, moves through thousands of energy channels called *nadis* that form a network in the body. When energy flow is restricted, it is believed that toxins gather in that area causing physical stiffness and pain.

THE BODY'S MERIDIANS

In Eastern medicine the body has 14 main meridians. Six are situated on each side of the body, one goes down the front and one goes down the back (see also page 10). Twelve of these are linked to internal organs and have an influence on them. The meridians are grouped in twos – one yin and one yang. Yin meridians are numbered from the lowest point, while

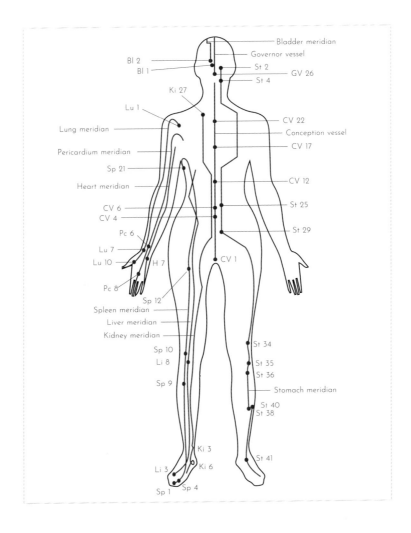

yang meridians are numbered from the top. The acupressure points are situated all along these meridians, and stimulating them can help cure certain ailments (see pages 53 and 68–69). Massaging your skin along a meridian route can help balance the body.

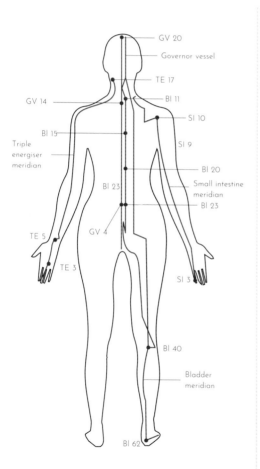

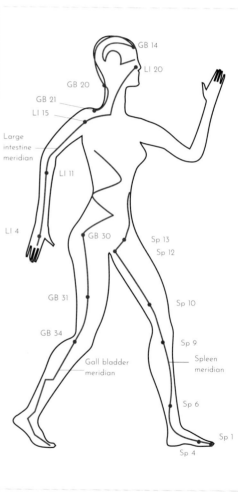

When hatha yoga (one of the main forms of yoga) is practised, three of the *nadis* are particularly important: the Sushumna nadi; the Pingala nadi (the sun channel); and the Idi nadi (the moon channel). Sushumna, the principal *nadi*, flows from the bottom of the spine to the top of the head. On its right-hand side flows the Pingala nadi, the active male channel that stimulates the physical body and transmits data from the left part of the brain, the rational side.

On the left-hand side flows the Idi nadi, the female channel that transmits consciousness to the body and sends messages from the right part of the brain, the creative side. Hatha yoga aims to balance these two life forces within the body.

THE AURA

To feel complete and function well, we all have a mind, body and spirit that need to be in harmony with one another. The philosophy of Indian and other Eastern therapies is to work towards achieving this harmony.

Many of us are good at worrying about the health of our physical bodies but we can too easily neglect our spiritual side. The aura is the subtle spiritual energy or electromagnetic field that surrounds a physical body. The more spiritually balanced we are, the wider our aura extends. An aura is oval in shape, with six coloured layers. The colours radiate from the major chakras: seven spiritual energy centres that penetrate all the layers. So the colours our aura projects change daily, showing the current state of our physical, emotional and spiritual health. There are three main layers of the aura:

> **The etheric body** is the layer nearest to our physical body (and they are closely interwoven) but it vibrates at a higher level. The etheric level helps to transfer prana from the universe to our physical body.

The astra/emotional body – the second layer – is wider and, because it is linked to the emotions, is often unbalanced. So, the colours of the aura change as we fluctuate from feeling wildly happy one day to being miserable or upset the next.

The mental body – the third layer – harbours our thought patterns; this is where they turn from thoughts into actions. It is from here that unpleasant thoughts about someone are projected to that person, which can be emotionally damaging all round. If we think negative thoughts, we attract more in return; conversely, if we think positively, positive thoughts will abound.

THE CHAKRAS

The word *chakra* is Sanskrit for 'wheel'; people who are psychic often see each *chakra* as a spinning wheel. Each *chakra* takes in energy from pulsating sunlight, and the Indians believe these spinning wheels are like lotus flowers, constantly opening and closing. There are seven main *chakras* in the body:

the red **Root chakra** at the base of the spine

the orange **Sacral chakra**, below the navel

the yellow **Solar plexus chakra** in the upper abdomen

the green (or pink) **Heart chakra** in the centre of the chest

the turquoise blue **Throat chakra** in the middle of the throat

the indigo **Third eye chakra** in the middle of the forehead

the violet **Crown chakra** on the top of the head.

Together the seven *chakra* colours make a rainbow, which in other cultures often represents the connection between our world and the gods.

Each *chakra* is associated with an emotional function and a body organ and is intrinsically linked to the endocrine system that controls the release of hormones in the body. So the chakras send energy to the endocrine system and vice versa.

When an imbalance occurs in a *chakra*, it either becomes smaller and spins more slowly, thereby affecting the health of the physical organs, or it spins faster and becomes larger, which can result in physical or emotional upset, such as an angry outburst or bursting into tears.

JUMP-START YOUR ENERGY FLOW

There are many complementary therapies that can work alone or alongside conventional medicine to treat a general lethargy or lack of energy in the body. With some techniques or holistic exercise regimes you can do them yourself (see Instant Energizers, pages 36–141) after learning the basics or following instructions; others, however, need to be performed by a qualified practitioner.

ENERGY-RELATED THERAPIES

Several therapies deal with correcting energy flow either through the body's meridians or *chakras*. With most therapies, a brief medical history is taken before diagnosis is made and any treatment begins.

Acupuncture – This powerful energy treatment is part of traditional Chinese medicine. A qualified acupuncturist performs the treatment. He or she makes a diagnosis by taking pulse readings and examining the face and tongue. For the treatment, fine sterilized needles are placed briefly in acupuncture points on the relevant organ meridian to remove a blockage or to stimulate sluggish *chi* flow.

Reflexology – This therapy is normally performed by a qualified reflexologist but you can do some simple treatments yourself (see pages 64–65 and 102–103). Although reflexology is linked to the Chinese meridian system, most therapists normally work with just ten vertical energy zones that start at the top of the head, branching out and stretching all the way to the fingers and toes; the main branches finish in the toes. In a treatment session, points are stimulated all over the feet or hands to boost energy circulation. Any blockages or imbalances can result in painful or slightly tender areas when pressed, and there may be some crystalline deposits that feel slightly 'crunchy' to the touch.

Feng shui – This Chinese art of furniture placement and *chi* flow in the home is performed by a feng shui consultant. He or she uses different techniques to achieve optimum energy circulation in the home and in work areas; consultants also advise people to clear out clutter, for example, as it causes debilitating energy blockages and stagnancy (see pages 94–97). Feng shui is often known as the 'acupuncture treatment of the home'.

Shiatsu – This Japanese therapy evolved alongside acupuncture and Chinese herbalism. Shiatsu literally means 'finger pressure', and practitioners use fingers, palms, elbows and other body parts to apply pressure to acupuncture points situated on the body's meridians to balance the energy systems.

Acupressure – Similar to shiatsu, acupressure involves pressure being applied to acupuncture points along the body's meridians to increase *chi* flow and remove blockages. Unlike shiatsu, however, only thumbs and fingers are used to apply pressure to the points. Nowadays, it is a popular self-help technique that anybody can use (see pages 53 and 68–69).

Reiki – This Japanese hands-on healing therapy means 'universal life force energy'. A reiki therapist provides treatment, but training is available to all. It works with both the meridians and the *chakras*, and stimulates the body's innate healing system. This relaxing treatment shifts blockages, thereby promoting a better energy flow throughout the body.

Yoga – This Indian exercise discipline uses different postures, meditation and breathing techniques to allow a positive *prana* flow to purify the body, mind and spirit. The full practice of yoga is best learnt from a qualified teacher but you can enjoy its benefits by learning a few exercises (see pages 50–51 and 124–125).

Chi kung or qigong – This ancient Chinese exercise system, from which t'ai chi originates, is also part of traditional Chinese medicine. In chi kung, a qualified practitioner teaches stretching, breathing and visualization exercises to get *chi* moving through the meridians inside the body, but you can practise a few simple exercises yourself (see pages 78–79).

Self-help techniques – In addition to acupressure, yoga and chi kung, there are other simple self-help techniques you can learn to promote harmony and good energy flow. Visualization is one such technique; for example, focusing on the colour that is lacking in an underperforming *chakra* can help to rebalance body energy. Meditation, massage, muscle-releasing and breathing exercises can also alleviate stress and tension in the body, mind and emotions, helping to release toxins – the body's major energy drainers. You can pick and choose from over 70 energizers in the Instant Energizers section, see pages 36–141.

We have become adept jugglers: trying to fit as many tasks as possible into each and every day.

2

ENERGY ZAPPERS

WHAT IS ZAPPING YOUR ENERGY?

In the hectic lifestyle of today we can too easily and regularly abuse our bodies. Constantly on the go and focusing on achieving as much as possible, we rarely make time for ourselves and often feel tired. We have become adept jugglers: trying to fit as many different tasks as possible into each and every day. We all strive for a work-life or family-life balance but few of us manage it; only rarely do we dedicate the time to nurture our physical, emotional and spiritual needs. There are many daily drains on our energy, and we need to recognize them so that we can avoid or resolve them.

PHYSICAL ENERGY DRAINS

As discussed earlier (see pages 6–7), to stay healthy with abundant energy, we need to eat a balanced and nutritious diet, get enough rest and sleep, and stay happy emotionally and spiritually. But when we are busy, or stressed, we can neglect our physical needs and our energy levels plummet.

Furthermore, we have the added problem of introducing toxins in the guise of alcohol, caffeine and nicotine into the body. Although we may rely on such stimulants, for example when we are trying to meet a deadline or entertain the kids on a rainy day, they actually work against us and upset the balance of our energy levels.

A SEDENTARY LIFESTYLE

Being inactive is an easy option when we are busy or overworked. Too many of us spend long hours every day working in one form or other without taking regular breaks, and we often drive everywhere (even short distances) rather than exercising by cycling or walking. But all our organs need a regular workout, particularly the heart, to thrive and make us feel good. A lack of physical activity reduces our energy levels, making us feel very lethargic and prone to mood swings.

Take action Do some daily exercise – just a short, brisk walk will work your heart and lungs and make you feel much more energetic and generally better in yourself.

ALCOHOL

This widely available stimulant is socially acceptable in many countries; many of us like to unwind from the day with a glass of wine or a beer. But alcohol is toxic to the body. Although enjoying a few glasses of red wine each week is thought to protect the heart, drinking to excess (more than 14 units for women, 21 units for men) strains the liver and reduces its ability to detoxify the body. Drinking too much alcohol also causes fatigue, dehydrates the body and brings on headaches. Furthermore, it disrupts sleep patterns and depletes the body of vital nutrients.

Take action Keep your alcohol intake below recommended limits and drink plenty of water every day (see pages 7) to eliminate toxic wastes. It is a good idea to have at least one or two alcohol-free days each week, if possible.

CAFFEINE

We mainly consume this powerful stimulant when we drink coffee or other caffeine-containing drinks, such as tea, cola drinks and hot chocolate. There is almost always enough time, it seems, to grab a coffee or tea to revive yourself. But drinking five to six cups of coffee on a daily basis is toxic to the body, wreaking havoc with the endocrine system. The stimulating effect induces the release of the hormone adrenaline, which promotes anxiety, restlessness, palpitations and insomnia. In addition, caffeine is addictive: you need to consume more over time to get the same buzz or lift, and when you try to cut down, the caffeine withdrawal brings on headaches.

Take action Stay more balanced by drinking caffeine-free alternatives, such as dandelion coffee or herbal teas, or limit yourself to one to two cups of coffee or tea daily.

NICOTINE AND OTHER TOXINS

Cigarettes contain nicotine, which is another strong stimulant. Inhaling the smoke from a cigarette may ease muscular tension and stimulate the senses, but it also activates the nervous system, releasing stress hormones into the bloodstream. Smoking just one cigarette speeds your heart rate and raises your blood pressure, putting strain on your cardiovascular system as the flow of oxygen in the blood decreases. Smoking is a serious health hazard: it greatly increases the risks of lung cancer, heart disease and stroke. Thousands of other toxins are introduced into the body through smoking, including carbon monoxide (a by-product of the smoke), which decreases oxygen levels in the blood and damages body cells, reducing the natural detoxification process.

Take action Stop smoking. You will have more energy within 24 hours as the carbon monoxide levels fall and oxygen levels normalize. After 1–5 years your risk of heart attack is halved. You can also try hypnosis, which has proved successful in helping some smokers to quit. If you're finding it hard to quit just yet, take a good multivitamin and mineral supplement daily to help counteract the depletion of nutrients.

EMOTIONAL ENERGY DRAINS

Apart from demands on your physical energy, you may also experience emotional drains that can come in many guises. Partners and family can wear you down with constant claims on your time. You may have certain demanding friends who zap your energy with selfish requests. At work, colleagues or bosses who undermine your position can lower your self-esteem. While in the home, entertaining the kids can sometimes make you feel isolated.

A LOVING RELATIONSHIP

The relationship you have with a partner can give you the most incredible energy highs and lows, depending on how well it is going. If you have a selfish partner and you seem to be the one that makes the compromises to keep the relationship going, there is an energy imbalance and you may feel unhappy and resentful. And if you constantly argue with a partner, your emotional energy will be at a low ebb.

Take action Talk through your feelings with your partner and suggest changes to bring the relationship back on an equal footing. And try to see if you can both work out why you constantly disagree. If a serious rift has occurred, joint counselling may well help to save the relationship.

CHILDREN AND AGEING RELATIVES

Both young and old can upset your emotional energy as they make demands on your time. Children can be easily upset by problems at school and young ones may have tantrums or upsets to get your attention. You may also find that older relatives, especially ones that are bedridden, think all your spare time should be spent with them.

Take action Conserve your energy by making a special time each day for your children to talk through their day with you; perhaps turn it into a story time for younger ones. Also, be realistic with needy relatives. It is a good idea to see them on a regular evening or weekend, so that they can look forward to the visit.

FRIENDS

Most of us have at least one friend who we would describe as self-obsessed or unreliable, or both. These 'energy vampires' will 'drink' you dry. You know the type. They phone you late at night with their current problems or crisis and never want to hear your news. Or they call you just as you are leaving to meet them to cancel with the weakest of excuses.

Take action Save your energy for yourself by limiting the amount of time on the phone to 'draining' friends. Reappraise your friendships. If one is over, explain why and move on. As you get older, your energy levels change and so will your friends.

COLLEAGUES OR BOSSES

People at work can sometimes be unsupportive, which can take its toll on your emotional energy and undermine your self-esteem.

Take action With an unappreciative boss, discuss a way to resolve your problems. Talk to unhelpful colleagues and see how you can work better together.

SPIRITUAL ENERGY DRAINS

Our spiritual needs are often low on the agenda. But if these are neglected, we will never achieve the perfect inner and outer harmony that we seek. Think about your life as it is today and study any areas where you are not happy that may be draining your spiritual energy. Watch your attitude, if you are constantly negative, your life will continue on that path. You may have a desire to paint or play an instrument but are not making the time to do it. Or, maybe your dream is to buy a property abroad, but you can't get round to doing the research on your chosen area. Perhaps you are in a mundane job that pays well, but you really desire to be a photographer or social worker.

Take action Make some regular time to connect to your inner self, as it harbours all your dreams and desires. Be positive and work to achieve your aims. Practise writing things down (journalling, see pages 128–129); you may be surprised at what you discover about yourself. Meditate (see pages 41 and 133) regularly in a quiet room to hear those inner messages that will keep you on the right path and let you fulfil your true desires.

*Be more selfish in the future and
give yourself more attention if you
want to feel really balanced again.*

3

FIRST STEPS

WHAT ARE YOUR DAILY ENERGY DRAINS?

One of the first steps is to recognize that your energy levels are being drained on a daily basis. The next step is to accept that you need to be more selfish in the future and give yourself some attention if you want to feel really balanced once again. Your family or friends may feel a little resentful initially when you decide to do this as your focus is taken from them to you. But this is the only way you are going to feel really good and have the energy you need to enjoy your life to the full.

Discover what your energy drains are by completing the following questionnaire on page 24 so that you can deal with them. You may well find that there are more emotional or spiritual causes than physical ones.

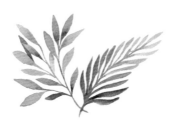

Complete the questionnaire below to find out how your energy is being zapped from your mind, body and spirit on a daily basis. Answer 'yes', 'no' or 'sometimes' to each question, noting down your responses.

1   Do you smoke more than 20 cigarettes a day?

2   Do you have a boss who never appreciates your work?

3   Are your constantly arguing with your partner?

4   Do you get anxious or worry about minor problems?

5   Are your drinking more than six cups of coffee daily?

6   Do you regularly not get enough sleep or sleep badly?

7   Are you stuck in a relationship that you don't know how to end?

8   Do you constantly feel that your life is going in the wrong direction?

9   Have you got achievable dreams that you are not putting into practice?

10 Are you always running yourself down?

11 Do you consistently work late?

12 Does your lunch often consist of a hurried snack such as chocolate or crisps?

13 Do you feel you give everything to your family but get little in return?

14 Is your computer, work space or home office full of clutter?

15 Do you get regular messages from your inner self, but choose to ignore them?

16 Are you longing to live in the country but stay in town?

17 Do you regularly get calls from friends who just offload their problems?

18 Are you often drinking more than 14 units (women) or 21 units (men) of alcohol a week?

19 Do you know that you are not in the right job, but are staying because of the money?

20 Are you often wasting your energy in senseless disagreements?

21 Is your normal attitude quite negative, do you view your life as 'half empty' rather than 'half full' in the glass analogy?

22 Are you always talking about making changes in your life, but then don't put them into practice?

23 Do you feel you have no time to take some spiritual space to meditate or do a yoga class?

24 Do you fail to make regular exercise a priority in your life?

25 Does your life seem empty right now, and you don't quite know why?

RESULTS

Now, add up your score. Give yourself:

2 points for a 'Yes'
1 point for a 'Sometimes'
0 points for a 'No'.

Total score = _____

Score of 35-50

Your energy levels are pretty depleted right now, so decide to make yourself your number one priority to refresh and restore them. Address any inadequacies or overindulgences in your diet and then look at improving your sleeping patterns. Next, take some time to analyse how you deal with family problems or unsupportive friends. Try to do some of the Instant energizers (pages 36-141) regularly to re-energize your life.

Score of 20-34

You are working hard but haven't totally neglected your overall energy levels. Still, they are lower than they should be, so look at any particular areas that need improvement. Make sure you have a nutritious lunch each day and that your alcohol intake is moderate. Work on any emotional drains in your life, such as a bad relationship. Follow your dreams and do a selection of the Instant energizers (pages 36-141) to give you the boost you need.

Score of 19 and under

Life is fairly under control for you; you have reasonable energy levels, but don't get complacent. You only need a difficult project at work or a crisis at home for them to start dropping. Look after yourself healthwise, and don't burn the candle at both ends. Keep physical, emotional and spiritual energy topped up by doing some of the Instant Energizers (pages 36-141) so that you stay happy and in balance.

PINPOINTING YOUR LOWS

Now you have completed the questionnaire on page 24, you will be more aware of which factors are responsible for your energy dips or lows. Note down any regular stimulants you use (see pages 19–20) and make a pact with yourself either to cut down on them or to give them up right now! Make a list of your current emotional drains and write down how you plan to deal with them.

ENERGY SLUMPS

Recognize which part of the day is worst for you. If you are a morning person, schedule important meetings or activities with children for the morning when you are at your most energetic. Note down the time when you start to feel tired and eat a high-energy snack (see page 8) half an hour before that time to even out your blood-sugar levels. If you are regularly exhausted and irritable by late afternoon, use a mid-afternoon boosting reflexology or breathing exercise (pages 86–105) to give you an energy boost. On the other hand, if you're a night owl who finds it difficult to wind down and get to sleep, cleanse your aura or do a clearing meditation before bed.

LONG-TERM LOWS

Spiritual lows can take longer to deal with as they often involve making life changes that take you out of your comfort zone. It may be that you want a more creative job or crave some 'you time' and a lie-in at the weekend, when your partner can deal with the kids. Whatever your goal, ensure you set time limits to achieving them. In the meantime, use mantras, self-affirmations and visualization exercises (see pages 36–141) to turn your goals into reality.

Write down a key affirmation that you can repeat aloud (at least ten times) to give you a boost when you are feeling low or insecure, or when you feel that life is not going your way. Choose your words carefully and make them positive. Try something like: 'I am a wonderful person and I am successful at everything I attempt'; 'I happily accept everything this new day brings me' or 'I have great health, love and happiness in my life'.

Build the larder gradually as you discover which
exercises and remedies work best for you.

4

THE ENERGIZER LARDER

CHOOSING REMEDIES

The exercises within the Instant Energizers section (pages 36–141) help you to maintain your energy levels during a normal day. To do many of these you require a selection of key items that you will use regularly, plus some others. Together these make up an energizer 'larder' that you can call on at any time when you feel your energy levels dropping. Build up the larder gradually as you discover which exercises and remedies in the Instant energizers section work best for you.

You may decide to buy several Bach or Bush flower remedies to even out your emotional lows. Rescue remedy, for example, can help panic attacks. Or if you are a tea drinker, you may want to buy fresh herbs and spices, such as warming ginger, to make various healing teas. The versatile and aromatic essential oils, which have the innate power to calm or revive the senses, will become an essential part of your larder. Start with the cure-all lavender oil and add others as and when you need them. You may also want to keep some incense and smudge sticks at home to cleanse negative and dull energy and bring a 'zing' back into the atmosphere. Finally, let the healing vibrations of crystals restore diminishing energy levels. Why not carry a nurturing stone, such as amethyst, with you – in your pocket or bag – to protect you. You will soon find the ingredients in your larder to be an indispensable part of your energy-balancing programme.

FLOWER REMEDIES

These natural liquid essences heal the mind, body and spirit. They harmonize any negative feelings stored in the subconscious mind. The essences are obtained when the healing vibrational quality or 'imprint' is extracted from certain flowers. This is normally done by the sun method: where the flowers are left in a bowl of water in strong sunlight, the resulting essence is poured into bottles half filled with brandy. Sometimes the boiling method is used: the flowers are simmered for 30 minutes in spring water and then decanted as before. The types used in this book are Bach flower remedies and Bush flower essences.

How to take flower remedies

With Bach flower remedies put 4 drops on your tongue or add them to a small glass of water 4 times a day. With Bush remedies, place 7 drops under the tongue, twice daily.

Bach flower remedy	Emotional cure
Elm p.59	Restores confidence in those who are overwhelmed with pressure from work or family commitments.
Hornbeam p.63	Gives emotional strength to face the new day for those who are mentally exhausted at the thought of too much work or too much to do.
Olive p.63	Replaces lost energy for those who are exhausted because of overwork or overexertion.
Rescue remedy (combination) p.63	Helps in emergencies or stressful events, such as taking a driving test, exam nerves or speaking in public, when there is emotional panic, loss of control and mental pain.
Willow p.63	Lifts the gloom and self-pity from an irritable and introspective pessimist who likes to wallow in misfortune.

Bush flower essence	Emotional cure
Alpine mintbush p.63	Gives joy and renewal to those suffering from mental and emotional exhaustion or from the weight of responsibility.
Calm and clear (combination) p.82	Encourages a person to relax and unwind when they feel overcommitted with no time for themselves.

continued opposite...

Crowea p.63	Balances and centres the individual who is worrying and feeling 'out of sorts'.
Dog rose of the wild forces p.67	Provides emotional balance for the person who fears loss of control.
Emergency essence (combination) pp.100–101	Helps ease distress and panic in someone who has suffered a shock.
Five corners bush flower p.47	Gives love and acceptance of self to those suffering low self-esteem.
Space clearing spray (combination) p.97	Creates a safe and harmonious environment where there has been a build-up of negative mental and emotional energy.

SMUDGE STICKS AND INCENSE

Smudge sticks are made from special dried herbs that are tied in bundles. When lit, their purifying scent recharges the atmosphere. When smouldering, sweet-smelling incense can brighten the ambience in a room. Choose one of these scents to use in the exercises in the Instant Energizers (see pages 36–141).

Incense	Effects of scented smoke (see p.134)
Cedarwood	Improves feelings of safety.
Cloves	Helps to boost concentration and lifts mood.
Jasmine	Relaxes the body for sleep and aids meditation.
Myrrh	Calms the emotions.
Sandalwood	Cleanses the atmosphere and enhances meditation.
Vanilla	Physically energizes but also calms the emotions.

Smudge sticks	Effects of scented smoke (see pp.122–123)
Rosemary	Cleanses stagnant atmosphere.
Sage	Purifies atmosphere on a deep level.
Sweetgrass	Drives away negativity.

ESSENTIAL OILS

These wonderful scented oils are aromatic essences that have been extracted from plants, flowers, trees, fruit, bark grasses and seeds. They have therapeutic psychological and physiological effects through their smell and through the skin. They can boost or relax our moods and promote healing in our bodies. About 150 essences exist, each with a unique scent and healing property. All have antiseptic properties but some also have pain-relieving, relaxing, stimulating and antidepressant qualities. It's a good idea to buy the multi-use lavender and tea tree oils first, then experiment with others (see table below and opposite) until you find ones that suit you.

How to use essential oils

Some essential oils can be used neat while others have to be diluted or mixed with a base oil. See pages 56, 63 and 108 for some examples of how to get the best from essential oils.

ESSENTIAL OILS HAVE THERAPEUTIC EFFECTS THROUGH THEIR SMELL AND THROUGH THE SKIN.

Essential oil	Properties
Basil p.108 (avoid during pregnancy)	Uplifting, harmonizing oil that increases concentration and clarifies thought processes.
Bergamot pp.43, 63 (use with caution in sunny weather)	Gentle, stimulating oil that is an effective antidepressant.
Camomile p.117	Relaxant that is antispasmodic, relieving tension headaches or an upset stomach.
Clary sage pp.43, 117 (avoid during pregnancy)	Antidepressant and relaxant that gives a euphoric feeling.
Eucalyptus p.97	Invigorating oil that cleanses the head and helps respiratory complaints.
Frankincense pp.56, 117	Calming, spiritually uplifting oil that soothes nervous conditions.

Geranium pp.108, 110, 117, 136 — Refreshing antidepressant that is good for nervous tension and exhaustion.

Ginger p.43 — Stimulates energy production.

Grapefruit p.117 — Tangy oil that gives an energy boost and alleviates nervous exhaustion.

Jasmine pp.108, 136 — Great fragrance that both relaxes and lifts anxiety, depression and lethargy.

Juniper p.131 (avoid during pregnancy) — Relaxing, purifying oil that can also refresh, particularly when run down.

Lavender pp.57, 108, 110, 117, 131, 136 — Versatile, relaxing oil that eases stress symptoms. It mixes with other oils and can soothe tension headaches, nervous digestive upsets and aid restful sleep.

Lemon pp.43, 117 — Cleansing, antiseptic oil that refreshes and boosts the immune system.

Lemongrass pp.56, 97 — Stimulating oil that cleanses and tones the mind and body.

Lime pp.108, 117 — Invigorating oil that can coax sluggish body organs into action.

Mandarin p.117 — Refreshing and cleansing oil that aids digestion and soothes heartburn.

Marjoram p.84 (avoid during pregnancy) — Calming and warming oil that releases tight muscles and reduces anxiety and headaches.

Neroli p.63 — Calming oil that lowers stress levels.

Orange p.43 — Revitalizing oil that is a tonic and raises the spirits.

Patchouli p.136 — Sensuous, relaxing oil that inspires the mind and lessens depression.

Pine pp.43, 117 — Cleansing oil that helps to lighten fatigue and tired muscles.

Rose p.133 — Fragrant, sensual oil that both soothes the emotions and eases muscular and nervous tension.

Rosemary pp.93, 97, 131 — Stimulating, cleansing oil that eases nervous exhaustion and mental fatigue.

Sandalwood pp.56, 136 — Heavy scented oil that is a relaxant and an antidepressant.

Tea tree p.43 — Useful cleansing, antiseptic oil that is very stimulating.

Ylang ylang pp.108, 136 — Soothing and sensual oil that is also good for stress, panic attacks, anxiety and depression.

HERBS AND SPICES

Herbal remedies have been used since ancient times to heal, and they still play an important part in healthcare in our lives today. Herbs (and spices) contain vitamins, minerals, trace elements and healing agents, such as tannins, butters and glycosides, that are beneficial to the body. Full of healthy nutrients, they can act as tonics or stimulants but can also impart a more calming influence. The antispasmodic and antiseptic qualities of some herbs calm the digestive system and boost immune function.

How to use herbs and spices

Fresh herbs are best to use when making the teas in the Instant Energizers' section so that you extract all the curative ingredients. See page 46 for the general principle of making herbal teas.

CRYSTALS

When hot gases and mineral solutions bubbled to the surface from the Earth's molten layer millions of years ago, the first crystals were formed. As the gases and liquids cooled, their atoms formed three-dimensional lattices, becoming the crystals we know today. Their crystalline structure enables them to absorb, strengthen and then transmit electromagnetic energy. This energy is used in crystal healing to balance the vibratory level of the aura, chakras and body cells. In healing, crystals can remove stress and negativity, dissolve blockages and bring harmony into your life. Initially, buy the stones for the main exercises in Instant Energizers and add in other suggested ones as and when you need them.

How to select crystals

Allow plenty of time in a crystal shop as the crystals you want will choose you. You will feel drawn intuitively to a particular stone, or when you pick one up you will feel an energetic connection or be comforted by it.

Herb or Spice	Uses	Properties
Ginger p.46	Warming and pungent spice that is best used fresh in tea.	Ginger aids fat breakdown and lowers blood cholesterol levels, speeding up digestion. It prevents nausea and is a good tonic encouraging blood flow, particularly in cold weather. It strengthens and heals the respiratory system.
Gingko biloba p.58	Ancient medicinal herb that can be drunk in tea to improve arterial circulation and increase memory.	It improves the use of glucose in the brain. It also increases mental alertness by stimulating the production of the brain's alpha waves.
Korean ginseng p.90	Root that is usually available as ginseng powder.	This stimulant increases energy levels, strengthens the immune system and decreases fatigue, thereby improving overall physical and mental efficiency.
Lemon balm p.58	Sweet-scented herb that has a pleasant flavour in tea.	Its antispasmodic qualities relieve muscle tension, alleviate nervous anxiety and help digestion.
Peppermint p.58	Herb containing menthol, which works as a carminative to reduce stomach tension or upset and feelings of nausea.	It has a fresh taste in tea, can aid concentration and can give you a 'lift' if you are suffering from exhaustion.
Rosemary p.46	Fragrant, aromatic herb that makes an all-purpose tonic as a tea.	Rosemary reduces the pain of a headache, can alleviate dizziness and strengthens the nervous system.
Sage p.46 (avoid if diabetic or pregnant)	Herb with a slightly bitter taste; add honey in tea to counter this bitterness.	Sage is a tonic that can also aid a griping stomach. It is also a relaxant that calms the nerves or overexcitement.
Green tea p.90	Eastern tea containing high levels of polyphenols and flavenoids that boost the immune system.	It has a strong antioxidant action that destroys free radicals that can increase the risk of cancer.

CLEANSING CRYSTALS

When you buy crystals they will have taken on the energetic imprint of the shop they have been in, so cleanse them thoroughly to re-energize them. If you use your crystals often to get rid of negative emotions, cleanse them regularly.

Water cleansing

Hold a crystal under running tap water to cleanse it. Focus on transmuting any negative energies into positive ones as the water is running over the stone. Leave it to dry in the sun.

Sunlight cleansing

Wash briefly under water and then leave on a sunny windowsill for 24 hours to renew its energy (avoid for amethyst and rose quartz as they are light sensitive).

SETTING YOUR INTENTION

You can utilize the energizing properties of crystals for many different forms of healing, but before you do this you need to make the crystal your own by setting an intention for its use, to 'switch' it on or 'tune' it in.

1. Hold the crystal in your hand, placing your other hand on top, and promise you will only use it for the highest good.
2. Become attuned to the crystal's energy; if you prefer, see a ray of white light connecting you.
3. Focus on the purpose for your crystal, whether it be for healing, meditation or cleansing, then dedicate it by saying out loud: 'I intend this crystal to help with ... (add your intention)'. Repeat it several times.
4. Keep a special crystal with you, in your car or by your bed at night.

Crystals	Uses	Qualities
Agate p.63.	Grounding stone that boosts self-esteem.	Promotes inner peace and improves perceptive skills.
Amber pp.76-77	Golden stone that heals the nervous system.	Promotes patience and brings wisdom and balance.
Amethyst p.130	Crystal that reduces physical and emotional pain.	Helps develop spiritual awareness and clear the aura.
Aquamarine p.83	Calming stone that reduces stress.	Makes the mind sharper and cleanses the Throat chakra.
Aventurine pp.60-61	All-round healing stone that promotes physical, mental and emotional wellbeing.	Enhances creativity and brings prosperity.
Beryl p.63	Crystal that encourages positive thoughts.	Alleviates stress and quietens the mind.
Bloodstone p.63	Stone that helps decision making.	Purifies the blood and grounds the body by cleansing the lower chakras.
Cat's eye p.63	Grounding stone that stimulates confidence and happiness.	Clears negativity from the aura and protects it.
Green tourmaline p.61	Powerful healing stone that opens up the heart chakra and promotes compassion.	Transforms negative energy into positive energy.
Jasper p.42	Nurturing and protective stone.	Promotes clear thought patterns and helps to balance the chakras.
Natural quartz p.91	Versatile crystal, which aids meditation, and amplifies the energy and the power of other crystals.	Reduces irrational fears and increases psychic abilities.
Rose quartz p.96	Wonderful healing stone that opens the heart.	Takes away negativity, heightens self-esteem and aids self-affirmations.

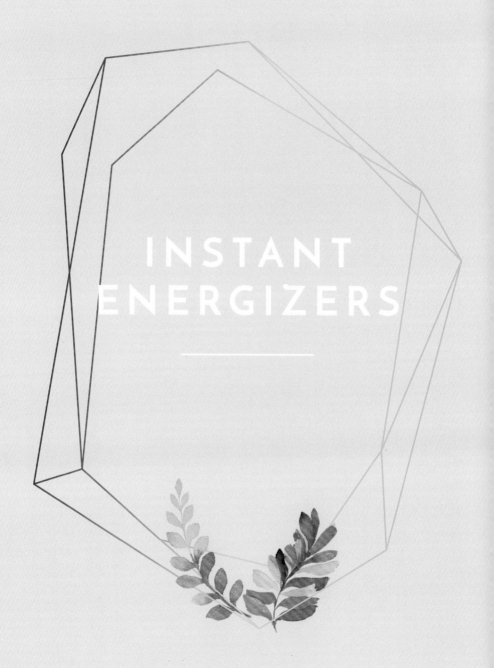

INSTANT
ENERGIZERS

WAKE UP FRESH

THESE EARLY MORNING HOLISTIC ENERGIZING EXERCISES
AIM TO GIVE YOU THE INITIAL ENERGY BOOST YOU NEED
- PHYSICALLY, MENTALLY AND SPIRITUALLY.

When you wake up in the morning your energy levels can be at a low ebb and you can feel sluggish and reluctant to begin the day. Your bodily systems will have slowed down for the long night's sleep and can need some encouragement to start working at full power again. Your mind may still want to linger in your pleasant dream world and not have the focus needed for the busy day ahead.

These early morning holistic energizing exercises aim to give you the initial energy boost you need – physically, mentally and spiritually. Clear and concentrate your mind with one of the meditative techniques, set your daily intent with an affirmation or work on both your body and your mind with some pre-breakfast yoga postures. The choice is yours; use one or two that seem appropriate. By practising these energizers regularly you will feel capable of handling all the challenges of the day ahead.

BREATHING FOR ENERGY

As your alarm sounds in the morning, it can be hard
to rouse yourself to get up from your warm, cosy bed
– and when you do get up you can feel lethargic and
find it hard to get going. Doing a morning breathing
exercise can give your body the stimulating uplift
it needs.

The importance of proper breathing is often
underestimated. As babies we instinctively breathe
deeply from our diaphragms, but as we get older
we become lazy and take shallower breaths from
the chest. When we inhale, oxygen from the air
is absorbed into our blood and is circulated to all
body cells and organs; when we exhale all the waste
carbon dioxide collected from the body is breathed
out. The more oxygen our blood receives the
healthier we are.

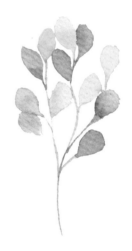

BREATHING DEEPLY

Take some deep breaths from your diaphragm to expand your
lung capacity and boost oxygen levels in your bloodstream, to clear
out toxins and to purify your internal organs before starting your
working day.

1   Stand upright with a straight spine or sit cross-legged on a mat
    on the floor. Breathe in deeply, through your nose, from your
    diaphragm, drawing air into your lower lungs.
2   As you expand your ribcage feel the air working up through your
    lungs until it reaches the top. Hold for a few seconds.
3   Slowly breathe out, through your nose, releasing the air first from
    the top of your lungs and then downwards. Repeat this deep
    breathing technique for about 5-10 minutes every morning.

WAKE-UP MEDITATION

Meditation is a wonderful technique to quieten your mind and bring inner peace; what is more, it is simple to learn. It helps you to leave behind all your fears, slows down your busy thought processes and separates you from your ego so that you can communicate with your subconscious mind that influences everything you do. Meditating for a short time each morning can reduce your stress levels and improve your overall wellbeing.

USE A MANDALA

Another technique to try is to meditate with a Tibetan or Buddhist mandala (a magic circle representing eternity). Take a colour copy from a reference book and place it in front of you. Focus on the central point of the circle as you start to meditate.

MEDITATE TO ENERGIZE

Practise this meditation for about 5-10 minutes every day. It won't take long to see its benefits: much more energy for the day and you will feel better able to cope with stress and life's hassles.

1   Place a lit candle in front of a yoga mat (or similar) on the floor, then sit cross-legged with a straight spine and with your heels together to help maintain your concentration and slow your mind.

2   Consciously relax all your body muscles, working through from the top of your head to your toes. Slow your breathing down, inhaling and exhaling deeply from the diaphragm.

3   Now gaze at the candle's flame. After about 60 seconds close your eyes, but hold the flame's image in your mind for as long as you can to quieten your mind. Now start to meditate, focusing on just one thought. As other thoughts intrude, just let them drift by.

4   Towards the end of your meditation, start thinking positive thoughts about the day ahead. See yourself enjoying yourself and being successful at everything you attempt. Slowly open your eyes; you are now ready to face any challenge.

REFRESH YOUR AURA

If you have a demanding day ahead, you may need some spiritual protection to help you cope. Everyone's bodies have a subtle spiritual energy field that surrounds them called the aura (see page 13). It has several layers and is filled with constantly changing colours that come from the light our bodies absorb. The aura also contains the seven main energy centres, known as the *chakras* (see page 14), that are situated from the groin area (the Root chakra) up to the top of the head (the Crown chakra). The aura reflects our emotional, mental and spiritual wellbeing, and its vibrational energies interact with our physical body, so they need refreshing regularly to stay healthy.

THE AURA'S VIBRATIONAL ENERGIES NEED REFRESHING REGULARLY TO STAY HEALTHY.

PROTECTING YOUR AURA

In addition to violet, white is another colour that links to the Crown chakra, our spiritual centre. Use it in this visualization exercise to fill your aura and protect it from daily negativity.

1 Sit cross-legged on a mat on the floor with a straight spine. Close your eyes and breathe deeply from your diaphragm.
2 Visualize a white light entering your Crown chakra on the top of your head; see it moving slowly through your body filling your organs and chakras until it reaches your feet. Sit for a few minutes and feel the warmth of this healing energy.
3 Now, see the white light expanding and forming a protective band around you. Feel its special power, then focus for a few minutes on your day ahead and slowly open your eyes. Repeat regularly to reinforce its powers.

ENERGY TIP

Hold a nurturing crystal, such as jasper, while you are doing this exercise.

AROMA CLEANSING

Once out of bed in the morning, your body can feel it requires a kick-start to get its circulation moving and to galvanize the body organs into action. Essential oils (see pages 30–31) are absorbed through the nose; their scents stimulating or calming the senses. They can also be taken in through the skin's pores, from where they are carried into the bloodstream, and quickly affect how you are feeling. Using a fresh, tangy essential oil, such as lemon, in your morning shower will give you a welcome uplift: cleansing your body, clearing your sleepy mind and elevating your spirit.

CREATING AN AROMATIC SHOWER

Choose a stimulating essential oil from the list (right) to make your morning shower an especially invigorating experience.

1 Mix 30-50 drops of your chosen oil in a 200-250 ml (7-8 fl oz) bottle of unscented shower gel; shake well. (Alternatively, mix 10 drops of your chosen oil in 15 ml of odourless vegetable oil. Dilute it half and half with water as you use it.

2 Run the shower until hot and steamy, step in and apply the gel direct to your body or pour some on a bath sponge and wash yourself.

3 Shower for about 5-10 minutes, allowing the aromatic scent of the oil to clear your head and inspire you for the day.

STIMULATING OILS

Citrus oils such as lemon, orange and bergamot are great tonics in the morning and are good skin cleansers to boot.

Clary sage oil (avoid if you are pregnant) encourages creativity.

Coriander oil brings inspiration.

Spicy ginger oil boosts mental clarity.

Pungent pine oil improves concentration.

Tea tree oil both cleanses and energizes.

GREETING THE DAY

Bringing fresh air into the home by opening windows in the early morning (and evening) is a wonderfully simple energizer to revitalize a home's atmosphere and release any stale energies from the previous evening. As the air pushes through, it takes with it moist kitchen or bathroom air, helping to avoid dampness and any fungal growth.

If your air quality is low, it affects how you feel and can deplete your auric field (see page 13). So flush air through your home daily for instant purification and cleansing.

BRINGING FRESH AIR INTO THE HOME IS A WONDERFULLY SIMPLE ENERGIZER TO REVITALIZE ITS ATMOSPHERE.

LET IN THE FRESH AIR

Opening windows to allow air into your home can transform the atmosphere from stale and stagnant to fresh and inspiring in a matter of minutes.

1 Your home needs to breathe. So each morning open one window at the front and one at the back for 10 minutes to allow a through passage of air.
2 Stand by the open window in the front and feel it brushing over your skin. Breathe in the air, feeling how it wakes you up and invigorates your lungs. Silently connect with the 'Spirit of the Air' and thank it for entering your home and removing any negative vibrations.

IONIZE YOUR HOME

Improve the quality of the air in your home with an ionizer, particularly in rooms where there are televisions or computers. An ionizer removes detrimental airborne pollutants containing positive ions and creates a negative-ion-rich environment in which we thrive. The ionizer brings an air quality similar to that by the sea or in a forest.

NEW DAY BEGINNINGS

Starting the day with a visualization exercise can reduce negative thinking and instil a new confidence in your capabilities. To make the most of the visualization first relax your body, which slows down your body organs and focuses your mind inwards, away from outside distractions. The visualization technique encourages 'right brain', more intuitive activity and the images that you will conjure up cancel out any destructive thoughts that the 'left brain', the ego or rational side, will try to engender.

VISUALIZATION TIP

If you are finding it hard to visualize, practise first by seeing yourself on your last enjoyable holiday; savour all the images, losing yourself in the happy scenes.

A BRIGHT NEW DAY

Practise this visualization technique to create the day you want and to achieve your planned objectives.

1 Sit cross-legged on a mat on the floor. Take several deep breaths from your diaphragm and then consciously relax your muscles, working from the top of your head down to your feet.

2 As your body relaxes, visualize your ideal day. Don't worry if initially you find this hard, keep concentrating and the imagery will come.

3 Start visualizing what you want. If, for example, you are giving a work presentation, see yourself smoothly coordinating the visuals with your talk. See how confidently you answer any questions. Feel and sense your power as your colleagues listen to your talk. Hear the praise as it ends successfully. Or perhaps you are a parent worrying about hosting your toddler's birthday party. See yourself happily organizing the food, controlling the party games and having fun.

4 Stay with these images for about 10 minutes, then slowly open your eyes; you are now ready for a successful day.

'GET UP AND GO' TEA

The natural healing ability of herbs is well known: they are an excellent source of vitamins, minerals and amino acids and can encourage healing in the body on a deep physical level (see page 32–33). Some herbs have properties that calm and sedate the organs after a strenuous day, while others are better for getting you going in the morning, invigorating the body and cleansing the blood. Making a herbal or spice tea (infusion) when you get up takes a little time but your body reaps the benefits of absorbing more of the healing herbal properties.

INVIGORATING ALTERNATIVES

Sage and rosemary both make refreshing teas. Infuse about 3 teaspoons of the fresh herb, or 1 teaspoon of the dried, in a teapot with the 2 cups of boiling water, as below. Leave for 10 minutes, strain and serve, adding the honey if needed.

GINGER AND LEMON TEA

A cup of this invigorating and fresh herbal tea benefits you from the properties of the ginger and the lemon. Ginger makes a fragrant, warming tea that promotes good blood flow, strengthens the respiratory system and boosts digestion. Meanwhile, the lemon offers you some antioxidant protection and provides vitamin C to increase your body's resistance to infection.

Ingredients

2 teaspoons fresh grated or dried ginger root
2 cups of boiling water
2-3 teaspoons fresh lemon juice
1-2 teaspoons fresh honey (optional)

Making the tea

1 Place the ginger in a china or glass teapot and add the boiling water. (Always make the tea in a non-metal teapot as metal can adversely affect the flavour of the herbs.)

2 Steep for 10 minutes, strain into a cup and then add the lemon, and honey if preferred.

THE POWER OF POSITIVITY

Beginning your day with a positive affirmation to suit your forthcoming challenges will surround you with creative energies. You may want to boost your self-esteem, deal with a work situation or overcome a niggling problem at home. Compose your own affirmations with words that really mean something, as they reflect what your mind truly feels. By constantly repeating your affirmation in your head, you embed that thought deep within your subconscious so that eventually it becomes reality.

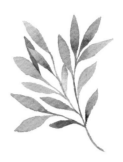

NEW DAY AFFIRMATION

Choose your affirmation to suit your day. Always use the present tense (or it won't work) and make sure your words support your aims. Write it down and say it aloud to enforce it.

1　Sit in a comfortable place or go for an early morning walk. Keep your affirmation short so that you can remember it.
2　Think of your affirmation, if it relates to self-esteem issues it may be something like: 'I love myself just as I am'; or maybe for a work situation: 'I am capable of communicating well with my colleagues'; or for a problem at home: 'I can resolve my conflict with the decorators'. Repeat your phrase 10-20 times to fix it in your subconscious.
3　Repeat the phrase throughout the morning as other negative emotions intrude.

ABSORBING

We take in colour from sunlight through our eyes, and to a lesser extent through breathing and through our skin. The eight colours of the spectrum – red, orange, yellow, green, turquoise blue, indigo, violet and magenta – affect our seven *chakras* (our spiritual energy centres), our organs and our endocrine system, which are all believed to be intrinsically linked.

Each *chakra* and body area has its own energy vibration. When any of these areas is not functioning well their vibration weakens. By treating these areas each morning with the colours they respond to, the body's vibrations – and the *chakras* – can be brought back in balance.

Interestingly, Western medicine now works with light and colour for people suffering from SAD (seasonal affective disorder).

OTHER WAYS TO TAKE IN COLOUR

You can also absorb colour from food. For example, indigo food such as blueberries, damsons or olives can be eaten to aid sleep and soothe an over-stimulated brain. Yellow food such as bananas, grapefruit and melons can boost the digestive system and reduce stomach problems.

ABSORBING COLOUR

Colour therapy (or chromotherapy) was first researched in the 1930s by the American scientist Dinshah P. Ghadiali. He discovered that the various colour vibrations our bodies receive from sunlight boost the functioning of organs, glands and emotions.

Both the physical body and its spiritual energy field (the aura) are part of the process, receiving and 'selecting' colour for the body. Ghadiali found that specific colours could help heal sick body parts. Turquoise blue, for instance, when held near or placed on the skin, helps resolve problems of the throat and lungs, improves functioning of the thyroid glands and encourages clear self-expression.

COLOUR BREATHING ENERGIZER

Colour can be breathed into the body through the air, so use this morning exercise to increase the energy in an under-performing *chakra*. Check the chart below if you're unsure which colour you need.

1   Sit cross-legged on a mat on the floor with a straight spine, keeping your shoulders down and back and your chest open. Do about five practice breaths, drawing the air in through your nose and down to your diaphragm. Hold each breath for about two seconds and then exhale slowly to a count of four.

2   Now close your eyes and meditate on the *chakra* colour that your body needs for this morning. When you see the colour in your mind, breathe it in on your next inhalation, and as you exhale, see it filling the relevant *chakra* area. For example, if you are visualizing red, see it flooding through your Root chakra around the top of your legs and pelvic area. Feel a shift in your energy as the blockage clears.

3   Work with breathing in this colour for around 10 minutes, and then sit quietly feeling any changes in your emotions or feelings. Do this exercise daily to correct *chakra* imbalances.

Crown chakra	Top of head	Spiritual feelings. Love of artistic pursuits
Third eye chakra	Middle of forehead	Intuition, clairvoyance, self respect
Throat chakra	Middle of throat	Self-expression, communication
Heart chakra	Centre of chest	Love and affection in relationships
Solar plexus chakra	Upper abdomen	Intellect and own power
Sacral chakra	Pelvic area	Creative urges, security and sexuality
Root chakra	Lower pelvic area	Survival and power

PRE-BREAKFAST YOGA

Yoga is a wonderful movement discipline that originated in India.

In Sanskrit the word 'yoga' means the union of mind and body. Hatha yoga is one of the physical forms and consists of a series of postures or asanas that help purify the body and mind. According to yoga teachings all bodily functions are controlled by an energy called *prana* (see page 9) that flows through channels called *nadis*. When you practise hatha yoga, *prana* moves positively through the body, clearing away toxins and promoting wellbeing.

Try out these simple yoga postures for 5–10 minutes in the early morning to increase the functioning of your body's organs, glands and nervous system. The postures also tone your muscles, increase your vitality and discipline your mind.

THE COBRA

This lying posture strengthens and tones the lower back, tightens the buttocks and boosts thyroid and adrenal gland function.

1   Breathe steadily while lying on your front on a mat on the floor, with your feet together. Place your palms under your shoulders next to your ribcage. Stretch your toes and point your chin towards the floor.

2   Inhale and lift your head off the floor, pushing up with your arms so that you look ahead. Keep your hip bones on the floor, breathe steadily and hold the position for about 10 seconds. As you exhale, lower yourself to the floor and return to Step 1. Repeat the movement.

3   Now, from Step 1, place your hands under your chest, this time with the palms facing inwards, and point your elbows outwards.

4   Inhale and pushing down lift your body off the floor. Look up, but keep your shoulders down and your hips just off the floor. Breathe steadily and hold for about 10 seconds. Exhale, then slowly lower yourself down. Perform 3-4 times.

THE TREE

This standing posture teaches you to balance, focusing your mind in the early morning and connecting your physical and mental energies.

1   Stand up straight and take 10 deep breaths from your diaphragm. Breathing steadily, balance on your right leg, then place the sole of your left foot on your inner right thigh. Push your right hip out, keeping your hips square.

2   Look straight ahead, concentrating on the wall in front of you. Don't worry if you wobble, just grip firmly with your foot. When steady, put your palms together and hold.

3   Now stretch your arms above your head, clasping your fingers and hold for about 5 seconds. Feel the energy move from your feet up to your fingertips. Slide your right leg down, repeat on the other side. Perform twice on each side.

MORNING MANTRA

Saying a mantra out loud can energize your mind, body and spirit. In this meditative technique Sanskrit (ancient Indian) words are chanted repeatedly to focus the mind.

Chanting a mantra creates a sound vibration that harmonizes the body and mind. Saying the chosen phrase over and over removes outer distractions, connecting you with your inner wisdom. It also benefits your body, working your respiratory system and promoting increased blood circulation and waste removal.

CHOOSING MANTRAS

Chant one of these mantras or find another that resonates with you.

'Om dum durgayei namaha'
Greetings to the female energy that protects us from negativity.

'Om gum ganapatayei namaha'
Greetings to the person who removes obstacles.

'Om namah shivaya'
No direct translation, but means: Greetings to the person I am capable of becoming.

MANTRA FOR A POSITIVE OUTLOOK

Chant this morning mantra regularly and see the beneficial changes in your mind and body.

1   Sit in the meditation position and relax your muscles (see page 41). Set your intent for the day

2   Choose your chant (see box above). You can start with a well-known one such as 'Om mani padme hum' (hail the jewel in the lotus), often shortened to 'Om'. You could use a word such as 'Peace', but chanting in another language is preferable as our words have many associations.

3   Close your eyes and chant your word establishing a rhythm as you do so and feeling a growing sense of peace. Chant for 5–10 minutes, then slowly open your eyes and become aware of where you are. You're now ready for anything.

AWAKENING ACUPRESSURE

If you lack energy in the morning, use this simple acupressure routine to perk you up first thing. Acupressure is an ancient Chinese healing therapy that uses finger and thumb pressure on acupuncture points on the body to stimulate the flow of chi (energy) through 14 main channels or meridians. Working on the points removes blockages and encourages the flow of sluggish energy. It differs from reflexology (see pages 64–65), which follows the recent concept of zones, rather than meridians. Allied to shiatsu, the Japanese pressure therapy, acupressure is ideal for self-treating as it is easy to learn.

MORNING ACUPRESSURE ROUTINE

This invigorating routine deals with a few of the body points, all of which are numbered and shown on pages 11-12. Work on these areas to boost your morning energy levels.

1   Stand or sit comfortably in a chair and start pressing gently with your thumb on point Sp 21 for 2 minutes to increase your vitality. This point is on the right side of the breast or chest.
2   Now to increase your energy, move on to the back of the arm and work your middle finger on points TE 5 (up from the wrist bone) and LI 11 (middle of elbow) for a few minutes.
3   To wake you up completely, rub your palms together to activate Pc 8 and then press them briefly on Ki 1 (not shown) on the soles of your bare feet.

MID-MORNING STRESS RELIEF

SPEND SOME TIME REFRESHING YOUR BODY'S ENERGY
LEVELS AND SEE HOW MUCH MORE YOU ARE NOW
CAPABLE OF ACHIEVING BY LUNCHTIME.

Mid-morning can bring a feeling of satisfaction for all the tasks you have already completed, but it can also bring some anxiety about what else you need to do for the rest of the day. Your physical energy levels may be dropping while your mind may still be 'buzzing' with your long 'to do' list.

This is an important time of day to stay in control and systematically plan the jobs to do next. Inevitably some stress is involved when you are busy, so aim to minimize it. The holistic energizers in this section can give you that physical and emotional boost. You can stimulate your senses with inspiring essential oils, drink a soothing herbal tea to balance your nerves, massage your temples and neck to ease tense and aching muscles or use a visualization technique to remove an energy block that is holding you back.

These energizers can be completed in a short break or a lull between tasks. Spend some time refreshing your body's energy levels and see how much more you are now capable of achieving by lunchtime.

STIMULATING THE SENSES

If you are having a busy morning, you may be feeling the pressure and in need of a quick energy boost. Rather than reaching for a cup of coffee, try this aromatherapy boost. Essential oils (see page 30–31) enter our bodies via our nose and sense of smell, so they can have an immediate and beneficial effect on our emotions. Keep some invigorating oils to hand so that you have an easy stress-relief remedy that will increase your concentration mid-morning, leaving you to carry on with renewed enthusiasm.

Rather than reaching for a cup of coffee, try this aromatherapy boost.

AROMATHERAPY TIP

If you plan to use essential oils regularly, it is a good idea to buy a plug-in electric burner that can be cleaned after use.

AROMATIC UPLIFT

Try out the different oils listed right to see which aromas appeal to your senses, increasing your energy and giving you mental clarity.

1 Put 4-5 drops of oil on a paper tissue or handkerchief. Hold the tissue to your nose and breathe in deeply for about a couple of minutes; feel the oil's instant effects.

2 Leave the tissue on your desk or kitchen table so that you can continue to inhale its aromas. Renew the oil hourly or as needed.

3 Alternatively, put the oil in a bowl of hot water and inhale deeply.

REVIVING OILS

Tangy citrus oils, such as lemon, orange and bergamot, are refreshing and clarify your thoughts.

Rosemary is revitalizing and balances the emotions.

Lemongrass oil acts as a refreshing tonic.

Frankincense soothes the nervous system and is spiritually uplifting.

Sandalwood calms and reduces stress.

TENSION RELIEF

When you are under pressure and working hard trying to keep everything running smoothly, tension from tight blood vessels in your head can build up, causing a throbbing headache in your temples. This can occur, for example, when you are looking after noisy children, or if you work in bad lighting conditions or spend too long in front of a computer. Lavender oil is a cure-all essential oil that can bring instant relief when applied to these tense areas. It induces calm and rebalances your emotions and energy, increasing *chi* flow to your Crown chakra – the spiritual energy centre (see page 14).

> **LAVENDER OIL IS A CURE-ALL ESSENTIAL OIL THAT CAN BRING INSTANT RELIEF WHEN APPLIED TO TENSE AREAS.**

HEADACHE EASER

Take a few minutes away from your busy day to do this soothing routine. Use lavender essential oil and work it well in to your temples to relieve pain or any energy blocks in the temples.

1 Sit comfortably in a chair and put a few drops of lavender oil on your fingertips; lavender is one of the few oils that can be applied to the skin undiluted.
2 Rub the oil in a circular movement around your temples and along your forehead for a few minutes until the pain or tension eases.

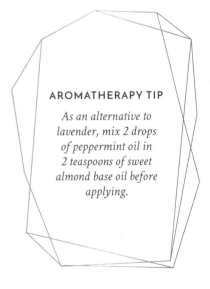

AROMATHERAPY TIP

As an alternative to lavender, mix 2 drops of peppermint oil in 2 teaspoons of sweet almond base oil before applying.

FORTIFYING TEA

Sipping a calming cup of herbal tea mid-morning can help you cope with a crisis, relieve your jagged nerves and balance your falling energy levels. Herbal teas are a healthier alternative to normal tea, which contains tannin and caffeine. The ingredients of some herbs (see pages 32–33 and 46) have the ability to act as a tonic and relieve irritability, nervous stomach cramps and anxiety. Making a tea from a fresh herb will give you the full benefit of its herbal properties, but if this is not possible use the dried herb or a herbal tea bag instead.

CALMING ALTERNATIVES

Lemon balm helps to calm the nervous system. It has relaxant and antispasmodic properties and can help irritability and restlessness.

Gingko biloba is a herbal stimulant and tonic that relieves headaches, improves blood and cerebral circulation, increasing short-term memory. Use it in tea bag form.

PEPPERMINT TEA

Peppermint makes a soothing tea that can boost your brain power, relieve headaches and clarify your thoughts. Its powerful menthol component can also help relax muscle tension or cramps in the stomach caused by stress. Drink this calming tea for added strength during the morning.

Ingredients

3 teaspoons of fresh peppermint or 1 teaspoon of dried peppermint
2 cups of boiling water

Making the tea

1   Place the peppermint in a china or glass teapot and add the boiling water.
2   Steep for 10 minutes, then strain and serve.

MIRROR POWER

Energetically, mirrors are believed to have great powers; in fact, in ancient times it was only people such as pharaohs and kings who were allowed to use them. In feng shui terms they are believed to double the positive energy of the space in which they are placed. So to instil some positive vibrations in your psyche to enhance the morning's successes (perhaps completing a project) or over-ride any failures (possibly arguing with your partner), say a carefully chosen, upbeat phrase while looking straight in the mirror. You are supposed to see your spiritual self in a mirror, so get in touch with your subconscious as you speak and feel your personal power increasing.

MIRROR WORK

Choose your phrase, then spend several minutes saying it in front of a mirror in the ladies' or men's room at work, in your work space or at home.

1 Take a few deep breaths to calm you, then look straight into your mirror and focus inwards. Connect with your spiritual image as you start saying your phrase out loud. It may be: 'My day continues well, I feel successful in everything I do', 'I am resolving this morning's problems' or 'I am a wonderful person, I can achieve anything'.

2 Repeat the phrase 10-20 times and feel a surge of spiritual vitality as you rebalance your energetic field.

ENERGY TIP

Take 4 drops of Elm Bach flower remedy (see page 28) on your tongue or mix in water and drink for extra confidence as you say your phrase.

BREATHING OUT STRESS

In times of stress a series of reactions is triggered in your body. As you panic the hypothalamus gland (your stress control centre) sets off a chemical chain reaction, triggering the release of the hormones adrenaline and noradrenaline, then cortisol into your bloodstream, activating all organs and cells. Your breathing becomes shallower, your heart races and your blood pressure rises, increasing blood circulation to the brain for quick thinking. You are now ready for action – to 'fight' or, conversely 'flee'. If this fight or flight response is followed by physical activity, this energy surge is used up and your body normalizes. But if you can't switch off, and still worry, you keep excess hormones in the body, putting pressure on your organs. By regulating your breathing you release pent-up tension and create inner harmony.

STRESS-RELIEVING TIPS

Do some deep breathing for a few minutes to calm you down. If you are feeling a bit out of control, put 4 drops of Bach flower Rescue remedy on your tongue to relieve your anxiety. Spray Bush flower Emergency essence into the atmosphere to calm any panicky feelings you are experiencing. Hold an aventurine crystal in your hands for about 10 minutes to balance your nervous system and blood pressure. Or use a tourmaline crystal to eliminate negative energy and strengthen your nervous system.

LETTING GO OF STRESS

When you know your body is under stress, take a few minutes to do this easy breathing exercise to ease your overworked organs.

1 Sit cross-legged on the floor with a straight spine and both feet flat on the floor. Keep your head in line with your neck and back. Focus on your abdomen and breathe in as you take your arms out to the side.

2 As you continue to breathe in and fill your lungs, lift your arms high above your head and look upwards.

3 Intertwine your fingers and continue stretching your arms. Breathe out forcefully, tilting your head back as you release all your stress and let your arms drop back down to your side. Repeat 5-10 times filling your lungs more deeply to clear all tension and re-energize your body.

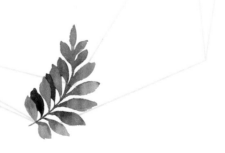

LETTING GO OF ANGER

If your morning is not going well and you are still seething or feeling very irritated after an argument with a colleague at work or because of an incident at home, take some time out to work on yourself. Anger is normal; it is a powerful agent of self-assertion and self-respect but it can become destructive if you are often having angry outbursts at the expense of other people. You may be projecting internal anger onto them because you are not handling your own stress well.

Suppressed anger is held as an energy blockage in the Solar plexus chakra (see page 14) in the abdomen. The blame and frustration here can be felt as a tight band in the stomach. Working consistently on releasing this pent-up anger will bring balance to this chakra, letting you deal with any challenging occasions.

ANGER RELEASE

This exercise can be done during a brief break at work or sitting in a chair at home. Work for several minutes, ideally 5–10 minutes, on the Solar plexus chakra until you can feel less tension in your stomach.

1   Sit comfortably on a chair with a straight spine. Close your eyes, if you can, and take a few deep breaths from your diaphragm.
2   Take your mind to your Solar plexus chakra, just below your breastbone in your stomach. See your anger there as a large, tight ball. Feel the anger, recent and longer-term, the hurt or pain; don't resist the feelings, let them flood your body.
3   Now focus on the ball and see it becoming smaller, and sense your anger diminishing and your stomach relaxing. Instil some feelings of empowerment in the chakra as you slowly come to. Do this exercise whenever you are losing emotional control. To cleanse sustained anger, do this exercise often until the ball completely disappears.

STRESS AND ANGER REMEDIES

Use the following Bach, Bush, essential oil and crystal remedies (see also pages 28–35) for anger control, and to help lower your stress levels.

Remedy	Emotion	How to use
Bach flower		
Hornbeam	Mental exhaustion	See page 29
Olive	Exhaustion with little strength or energy	See page 29
Willow	Irritable and wallowing in self-pity	See page 29
Bush flower		
Alpine mint bush	Mentally and emotionally drained	See page 29
Crowea	Emotionally out of balance	See page 29
Essential oils		
Bergamot	Feeling stressed out	Put a few drops in an oil burner or use on a tissue
Neroli	Stressed and anxious	As above
Rosewood	Angry and irritable	As above
Crystals		
Agate	Bitterness and inner anger	Hold crystal in hands for 5 minutes and ask for cleansing
Beryl	Stressed and lacking courage	Place on Solar Plexus chakra and draw in healing energies for 5 minutes
Bloodstone	Feeling toxic and lacking energy	As Agate
Cat's eye	Feeling negative and lacking confidence	As Beryl

REVIVING REFLEXOLOGY

Performing a short reflexology routine on your hands or feet in the middle of the morning can work wonders for flagging energy levels as well as alleviating any taut muscles in your shoulders and back.

This ancient therapy was first introduced into Britain in the late 1960s. Also known as zone therapy, reflexology is a treatment where pressure is applied to points and nerve endings on the feet and hands to encourage healing and good energy flow. As in acupuncture, the points are linked by ten 'reflex' zones to muscles and organs in the body, so that when stimulated the entire zone benefits. By massaging different points you can clear energy blockages and improve overall health. Ideally, take a break to do the reflexology, but if this is not possible you can work on a foot with one hand while still working.

A SHORT REFLEXOLOGY ROUTINE CAN WORK WONDERS FOR FLAGGING ENERGY LEVELS.

REFLEXOLOGY TECHNIQUES

Most reflexology points are worked on with the fingertips and the edge of the thumb:

Thumb- and finger-walking – Flex your thumb or finger as you slide it forwards in a similar movement to that of a caterpillar.

Rotating on a point – Keep either your thumb or your index finger on one point and rotate it slightly to activate the point.

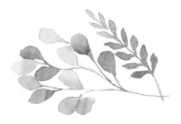

INVIGORATING REFLEXOLOGY ROUTINE

Increase your energy flow and release the tension from your shoulders and back by spending a few minutes stimulating the points described below. Use both your hands and your feet to activate the relevant points.

1 A short reflexology routine can work wonders for flagging energy levels.
2 To release the stiffness in aching shoulders, press and knead the fingers of both hands across both the top and the sole of each foot, about 25 mm (1 in) from the toes.
3 Pinch, press and gently rotate your thumb to the count of five on the shoulder point, which is located between the base of the fourth and the fifth toes.
4 Alternatively, work your hand between the bases of the fourth and the fifth fingers.
5 To get the energy flowing, finger-walk your thumb or finger down the spine area, which is the bony ridge of your hand from the side of your thumb down to the wrist.
6 To ease aching back muscles use four fingers to knead or finger-walk horizontally along the bony ridge of your hand, pressing slightly harder on any sore areas. Finish with some soothing strokes down the hand over the spinal area.

FREE-FLOWING ENERGY

Mid-morning can seem quite late in the day if you have started work at a breakfast meeting or if you have been busy with children since the early hours. You may be feeling down and not quite right. You can sense that your energy is depleted and that a certain part of your body is causing the problem, but you don't know exactly where. You may even feel a bit shaky or queasy. These sensations are often an emotional imbalance causing an energy block in your body (see the *chakras* page 14).

Use the following exercise to discover the location of your blockage so that you can treat it with healing energy and continue your day with renewed vigour.

REMOVING ENERGY BLOCKS

After scanning your energy field (see opposite), try this visualization for about 5 minutes or so when you have a quiet moment at work or at home.

1   Sit comfortably in a chair with a straight spine. Close you eyes and breathe deeply from your diaphragm to calm you.
2   As your breathing slows, imagine yourself sitting in a field in mid-summer, the sky is completely blue but there is one dark cloud obscuring the sun. Now see this same imagery inside your body with the dark cloud being your blockage in your throat or stomach, for example.
3   Slowly see the dark cloud getting smaller and smaller as the sun starts to break through, feel its warmth as it breaks up the last pieces of the cloud, removing your blockage. Now let your whole body be filled with the healing yellow light. Sense your body relaxing as your energy starts flowing well again. Come to, energized and ready to tackle anything the rest of the day throws at you.

SCANNING YOUR ENERGY FIELD

Learning to scan your body to discover energy imbalances or blockages takes some practice, but you will soon get to know your body. Always scan your body before doing the visualization opposite.

1   Take off your watch and any rings or bracelets. Rub your hands together, then put your hands palms up and see if you can feel any 'tingles' – this is you own electromagnetic energy field.

2   Hold your palms facing each other, and then curve them slightly as if they were holding a soft ball, about the size of a football. Move this imaginary ball back and forth between your palms for a few minutes and sense the energy flow that exists between your hands.

3   Now your hands are sensitized, start to scan your body. Hold your hands out about 25 cm (10 in) in front of you, palms inwards and move them down your body from your head to your feet to find any blockages. Balanced areas usually feel warm; hot and tingly areas can indicate a painful or injured area, cold areas indicate an energy blockage. Note where your blockage is so that you can work on it (see opposite).

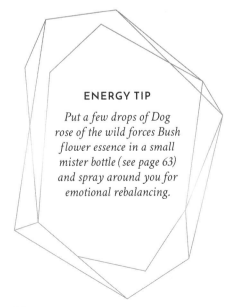

ENERGY TIP

Put a few drops of Dog rose of the wild forces Bush flower essence in a small mister bottle (see page 63) and spray around you for emotional rebalancing.

HEALING ACUPRESSURE

This soothing acupressure routine can help to release any pent-up anxieties, release muscle pain, lower your stress levels and alleviate any mild depression that you are suffering.

As mentioned earlier (see page 53) finger or thumb pressure is used in acupressure on different acupuncture points to balance the body's energy flow. To reduce any symptoms of stress, it is necessary only to touch a few points to gain some relief and a calmer attitude that lets you cope with the rest of the day.

SOOTHING ACUPRESSURE CAN HELP TO RELEASE ANY PENT-UP ANXIETIES AND LOWER YOUR STRESS LEVELS.

PRESSURE PRINCIPLES

You can press into points with either your index finger or, for increased pressure, your thumb. Don't dig too hard so that it hurts, just massaging or stroking the area can be sufficient. With a tender area, massage with one finger in circles gently above and below it, before pushing the point itself very gently.

MID-MORNING ACUPRESSURE ROUTINE

In a quiet moment, work on the numbered points below for a few minutes, or until you feel your symptoms easing. See pages 11–12 to identify and locate body points.

1   Sit comfortably in a chair, lift up your left lower leg and rub your fingers up and down the fleshy outer sides of the leg to stimulate the Spleen meridian and point St 40 on the Stomach meridian. This can help to 'ground' you. Repeat on the other leg. Also work with thumb pressure on Lu 7 on your inner wrists and Lu 10 on the fleshy part of your thumbs to release stagnant energy that can make you feel down and free any blocked emotions.

2   To reduce tension and anxiety symptoms work with thumb pressure on Li 3 (between the second and big toes) on the Liver meridian, Li 4 – the great eliminator – (between the first finger and thumb in the fleshy part at the end of the thumb), the Large intestine meridian and calming H 7 (below the bony prominence of the wrist on the outer side of the little finger) on the Heart meridian.

3   Stretch out your spine and breathe deeply from your diaphragm as you touch the 'sea of energy' CV 6 on the Conception vessel, two finger-widths below the navel to bring energy down and alleviate muscle tension, or while you gently massage the heart point CV 17. When you are worried, rub your stomach with the base of your palm, clockwise and anticlockwise to relax the muscles.

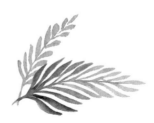

LUNCHTIME REVIVERS

JUST WALKING OUTSIDE CAN HELP YOU REFLECT ON
WHAT YOU HAVE ACHIEVED IN THE MORNING.

Taking some time for yourself over lunch gives you a chance to clear your head and lose the worries of the morning. Get away from a computer, phones or commitments, turn off your mobile and escape outside so that your body and soul can reconnect with the soothing rhythms of nature.

Doing these exercises outside replenishes your mind and emotions and inspires you to continue the afternoon with enthusiasm. Hug a tree to receive its wise and balancing energies or walk barefoot and sense the power of Mother Earth. But don't worry if you have to stay inside, you can still reduce the pressures of the morning by doing a mini Indian-type head massage to banish any irritations or the visualization exercise to dispel any tensions.

Find the energizer for you. If possible do two each day, and see how much more motivated you feel when you return to your afternoon tasks.

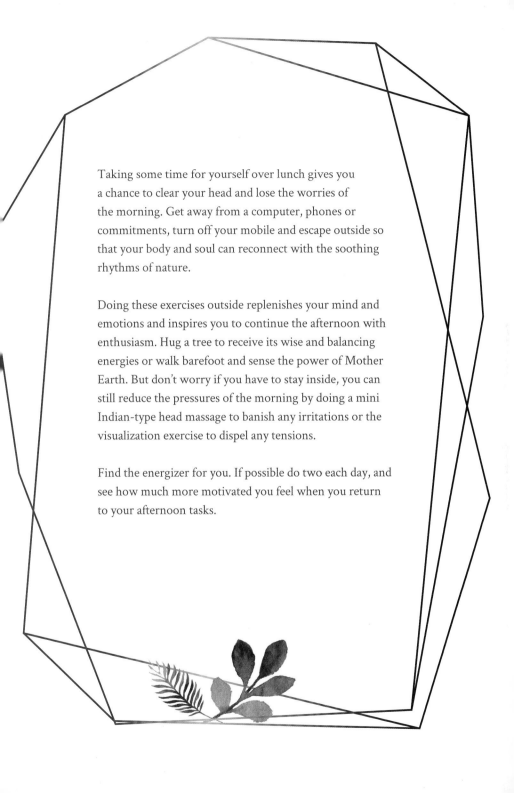

WATER CLEANSING

Leave behind the cares of the office or trials of home life to do this outside water meditation, which will cleanse your body of any worries.

Water is believed to have special purifying and sacred powers, and was often used in native healing ceremonies to soothe the spirit of an injured person. Today, water still retains the essence of a nurturing and healing energy. Looking into the hidden depths of water is supposed to be a source of wisdom, so sitting by a pond, lake or river can give you the chance to meditate and reflect on your life's purpose.

If you meditate by water regularly at lunchtime, you will soon see how its purifying influence helps you cope with your daily stresses. If there is no water nearby, sit in a green space and visualize a vast expanse of water in your mind first, before starting the meditation.

WATER IS BELIEVED TO HAVE SPECIAL PURIFYING AND SACRED POWERS.

WATER FEATURE

If getting outside is difficult and you want to try water meditation, place a water feature on your desk or on a table at home. Ideally, buy a small fountain with running water or one that runs over pebbles. Alternatively, place some chosen pebbles in the bottom of a square vase and fill with water. Gaze into the flowing or still water to inspire your meditation.

WATER MEDITATION

Practise this meditation for about 10 minutes, losing yourself in the nurturing influence of the water.

1   Sit comfortably on a bench in a park by a lake, on a riverbank or on the seashore on a calm day. Gaze into the water and start to slow your breathing, taking deep breaths from your diaphragm.

2   Feel the serenity and peace of the water and sense how it welcomes you. As you start to lose yourself in its infinite depths, let its cleansing presence wash through your mind, removing any anger, irritation or criticism that has occurred in the morning.

3   Let out any annoyances or emotional upsets and watch as they float away on the water. Feel positive thoughts about your capabilities entering your mind. See the challenges of the afternoon as a detailed list but only sense calm when you look at it. Slowly come to (or open your eyes) and return to face the afternoon with your energy levels recharged.

ENERGY TIP

Water stimulates and encourages the flow of chi, so put a running water feature on the southeast corner (your wealth space in feng shui) of your desk or on a table in this area of your living room to encourage success.

CONNECT WITH THE EARTH

Taking time out at lunchtime to go outside and walk barefoot on the ground, connects you with nature and inspires your soul.

In the Western world, most of modern life is spent indoors in artificially lit and centrally-heated buildings. We spend so much time indoors that we are rapidly losing our connection with the seasons and the natural energies of the planet.

Our bodies are familiar with the 'grounded' and strengthening electromagnetic fields that emanate from the earth, but by wearing shoes all the time we are losing our sensitivity to this powerful energy.

Walk barefoot outside during the summer months and whenever you can in the home to reinforce your connection to this ancient healing energy source.

ENERGY TIP

Bring some earth energy inside. Keep a smooth pebble on your desk or on a windowsill at home. Buy one or preferably find one in a favourite place, perhaps by a river or the sea, so that you transfer the vibration of that beautiful place inside.

MOTHER EARTH

Ancient civilizations that lived and worked on the earth, thought of Mother Earth as the fertile provider for all. There was a deep sense of partnership, of living with the earth. Pre-Christian peoples, such as the Druids, were so in tune with nature that they built sacred buildings in accordance with the elements, and where they felt strong earth energies. This connection is being revived today by people supporting the Gaia theory that what we do to the earth, we do to ourselves.

WALKING BAREFOOT ON THE GROUND CONNECTS YOU WITH NATURE AND INSPIRES YOUR SOUL.

_____

BAREFOOT WALK ON GRASS

Go barefoot walking in a local park or on your garden lawn for about 10 minutes to strengthen you in the middle of the day.

1   Take off your shoes and any socks or tights and stand upright on the grass for a few minutes to connect to the earth's energies. Deeply breathe in the fresh air and curl your toes a couple of times in the grass to feel its texture and freshness.

2   Now walk along the grass enjoying each step, let the sweet smell of the earth fill your nostrils and seep into your lungs. Feel the chatter of your mind quietening, and any tiredness or tension leaving you as you become at one with nature's grounding and creative source.

3   Walk for about 5-10 minutes and sense the profound intimacy of being in touch with Mother Earth. Put your shoes on and return inside feeling revitalized for the afternoon ahead.

EMBRACING TREE ENERGY

It may sound a bit wacky to escape outside at lunchtime to go and hug a tree, but the harmonizing and balancing energy they give out can calm and refresh you. The solid strength of an old tree is very protective and reassuring, and, once again, very 'grounding', especially if your morning has been challenging or chaotic.

The ancient Greeks worshipped trees as they thought they were oracles of the gods, while many Native American tribes consider them to be sacred and would never deliberately cut them down.

Trees put down deep roots into the ground; so spending some time with them can reassure you and literally 'bring you right back down to earth'.

THE SOLID STRENGTH OF AN OLD TREE IS PROTECTIVE AND REASSURING, AND VERY 'GROUNDING'.

SHAMANIC HEALING

Shamans or healers of Native American tribes often used the roots of a tree or a tree stump as a pathway or gateway as they 'journeyed' (a deep visualization technique) from ordinary reality to the lower worlds in the spirit realm – the tree acted as the transition between the two worlds.

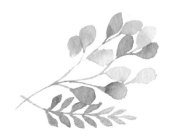

TREE HUGGING

Choose a quiet place and stand and hug your chosen tree or sit with your back next to a tall strong tree for at least 10 minutes; let its healing energies bring you mental clarity and emotional serenity.

1 Sit on the ground behind your tree and wrap your arms around it. Alternatively, sit with your back straight up against the tree.
2 Close your eyes and take some deep breaths from your diaphragm and relax your muscles. Remove your shoes, and put your feet flat on the ground so that you are 'rooting' yourself in the earth.
3 Now let go of any negative thoughts, anger or resentments that have been held for a while or that have built up during the morning. Visualize them being soaked up by the earth and dissipated by its healing energies.
4 When you have released all the negativity, imagine this healing energy coming up through the soles of your feet, working its way up through your legs, stomach, chest, through your arms, until it goes out through the top of your head. Sense this energy as a 'tingling' feeling.
5 As you absorb this earth energy, let some pure golden, protective universal light travel your body through the top of your head down to your feet. Keep breathing deeply as you feel the warmth of the two energies mixing. Slowly open your eyes, sensing how much more balanced and harmonized you feel. Let go of the tree, thanking it and Mother Earth for their loving, healing energies. If you want, leave a small token, such as a coin or a small crystal, as a thank you to your tree.

CRYSTAL TIP

Put a piece of amber in your pocket as you hug your tree to facilitate the balancing of your energies and calming of your nervous system.

LUNCHTIME CHI KUNG

Chi kung or qigong literally means 'training the breath' or 'energy cultivation' (*chi* or *qi* means energy and gong means cultivation).

It evolved in China many centuries ago and it is the exercise movement from which t'ai chi originates. There are many forms of chi kung but the main aim of 'internal' chi kung is to manipulate the flow of chi inside the body to stimulate healing. The 'hard' martial art forms of this art are t'ai chi or kung fu, while a 'softer' form just works with moving chi internally. Aerobic conditioning, meditation and relaxation are all part of chi kung, as there is no extreme exertion it is suitable for all fitness levels.

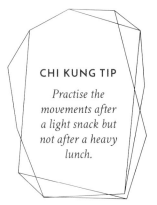

CHI KUNG TIP

Practise the movements after a light snack but not after a heavy lunch.

WARM-UP EXERCISES

Do a few of these warm-up exercises for several minutes before starting The Shower of Light routine.

1　Stand with your feet a shoulder-width apart. Start to bounce up and down on the balls of your feet.

2　Start to swing your arms back and forth energetically to get rid of stale air and toxins in the lungs. Inhale as you go up on your toes with your arms up and exhale as you go down and swing your arms behind you. Also swing from side to side to warm up the muscles.

DO THIS EASY CHI KUNG ROUTINE AT LUNCHTIME IN THE FRESH AIR TO REMOVE ANY HARMFUL CHI FROM YOUR AURA.

———

THE SHOWER OF LIGHT

Perform this routine for about 10 minutes to fill your body with new vibrant energy.

1   Stand with your feet shoulder-width apart. Turn your palms outwards, breathe in and slowly raise up your arms in front of you.
2   Continue raising your arms up to your head height, keeping them slightly curved in shape.
3   When you arms are right over your head, imagine fresh *chi* filling your palms from the sky.
4   Breathe out, slowly bringing your arms down the front of your body, this time with your palms facing inwards.
5   Keep breathing evenly and continue to bring your arms down until they reach your navel. As you do this movement, visualize the fresh *chi* flowing down your front, your back and sides through the body's meridians (see pages 11–12), flushing out any negative *chi*. Bring your hands back to your side, and repeat the sequence about 6 times.

CLEANSING BREATHING

Having a break at lunchtime often gives you a chance to go outside in the fresh air to revive you and lift any tiredness you are feeling.

As was discussed earlier (see page 40), breathing deeply and slowly improves your body functions and increases your general wellbeing. Check your breathing throughout the day; it is very easy to breathe shallowly if you are stressed. Stop to take a few deep breaths, and maybe yawn and stretch out your arms to get in touch with your body.

Cleansing breathing, preferably out in the open air, can release any anxieties or disperse any stagnant energy from the morning into the outside atmosphere.

BREATHING TIP

Bring yourself into the 'now' by breathing in future dreams and breathing out negative aspects of your past.

BREATHING OUT STALE ENERGIES

Perform these breathing exercises for 5-10 minutes and let the new energy you absorb revive your body and spirit.

1   Sit comfortably outside or in a quiet space inside. Take a deep cleansing breath through your nose, pulling the breath right up from your feet through your body. Breathe out forcefully through your mouth, blowing out any stagnancy or anxiety held inside. Repeat for several minutes.
2   Now, breathe in deeply and imagine a fountain in your lungs that rises up, getting taller and taller until it overflows through the top of your head as you exhale. Repeat for a few minutes until you feel energized.

LUNCHTIME SINGING

After a busy morning where it feels like you haven't stopped since you got up, you may be feeling emotionally drained. If you can make time and find a quiet space outside, or inside, to sing you will ease any jaded emotions and bring some joy back into your soul.

When you sing you also improve the resonance and flexibility of your speaking voice. As you sing confidently, you naturally raise your spirits by breathing more deeply and releasing any anxieties that you are holding inside. You also benefit from the higher levels of oxygen being absorbed into the bloodstream. Our body cells and organs react to different sound vibrations, which can change when an area is under stress, so singing can help restore these vibrations to their normal level.

WHEN YOU SING YOU ALSO IMPROVE THE RESONANCE AND FLEXIBILITY OF YOUR SPEAKING VOICE.

UPLIFTING SINGING

Find a quiet space, outside if you can, where you won't be disturbed and sing your heart out for 5-10 minutes. If it's difficult to find a quiet space, why not sit in your car?

1   Choose a favourite song that you can remember well. Start to sing softly at first until you get into the natural rhythm of the song.
2   As you become more confident, you will breathe in deeply and sing more loudly; at the same time, you can sense how any tension in your chest or stomach simply dissolves. Feel the vibrations coursing through your body, giving you a feeling of joy and happiness.

CREATING BLISS

Even with only half an hour to spare at lunchtime, you can do this visualization exercise outside or inside to take you to a favourite place and leave behind the morning's upsets.

The visualization technique consciously uses your imagination to create attractive and positive imagery to heal negative thoughts or to make changes in your life. If you think of the stress symptoms you experience when you worry, the opposite effects are achieved with visualization. The strong positive images the brain receives brings serenity, over-riding any destructive thoughts. The body releases tension and positive physical effects take place.

ENERGY TIP

Spray some Calm and clear Bush flower combination essence into your aura (see page 29) before your visualization to help you wind down.

INDUCING CALM

Spend 10 minutes on this visualization technique to visit your special haven and find peace.

1 Sit comfortably and relax. Close your eyes and think of a favourite scene where you always feel at peace. It may be on a beach from a dream holiday, by a lake or river or even in your garden.
2 Now take yourself to this place and lose yourself in the environment. See the colours, hear the wildlife, smell the scents. Feel the tranquillity of the place rejuvenating your body and resolving any problems; see hassles just drifting off into the atmosphere.
3 Slowly open your eyes and come to, knowing you can return here at any time to feel this calm and to deal with any worries.

CRYSTAL CLEARING

For thousands of years crystals have been used for healing and protection (see pages 34–35). Every *chakra* (see page 14), cell and organ in our body is believed to vibrate at its own frequency. If these become unbalanced or upset, illness can result. By setting a mental intent you can send healing energy (directed from the universal life force) into a crystal so that it emits the electromagnetic vibrations needed to restore the healthy functioning of a *chakra* or body part.

Working with an aquamarine crystal regularly at lunchtime will help you speak out and give your mind a therapeutic workout.

CRYSTAL HEALING FOR MENTAL CLARITY

Work with a cleansed aquamarine crystal (see page 35) for 5-10 minutes to clear your mind and restore any blocked communication.

1　Sit comfortably in a chair, close your eyes and hold your crystal for several minutes. Tune into its energies, having already set its main intent (see page 34). Ask the crystal to clear your mind of any distractions and fears.

2　Now hold your crystal for a few minutes over your Throat chakra in the middle of your throat and ask for any communication problems to be removed. Open your eyes and thank your crystal for its healing energies.

CRYSTAL TIP

You can also cleanse your crystal by smudging. Light a herbal smudge stick (see page 122), hold over a flameproof dish and waft the purifying smoke over your crystal; you can cleanse several crystals together in this way.

HEALING HANDS

If you don't have time or can't get outside at lunchtime, you can still boost your energy levels by using the power of your hands.

Your hands can be used for two different healing routines: by massaging your hands, you can relieve any aches and strains in your fingers; by working on your head with strong fingers, you can release tension that has built up during the day.

OILS TO USE

Marjoram essential oil.

A proprietary base oil such as grapeseed, sunflower or safflower oil.

LUNCHTIME HAND MASSAGE

The hands respond as well to massage as the rest of the body. By massaging them you can get the blood flowing and shift any tension in the muscles and joints caused by rigid or repetitive movements. Try this relaxing massage with essential oils to ease aching fingers when you have been typing on a keyboard all morning or driving for a long time without a break.

Work on your hands using these circling, kneading and stretching techniques for 5-10 minutes to reduce nagging aches and pains.

1   Mix 3 drops of marjoram essential oil to 3 teaspoons of your base oil in small plastic bottle.
2   Sit comfortably in a chair. Rub some massage oil into your right hand. Breathe in and out gently as you squeeze out tension between each finger on your left hand with your right thumb and fingers. Then press and rotate your right thumb into the back of your left hand, working over the whole area.
3   Turn your hand over and repeat the circles on your palm, kneading the hand with strong strokes to release contracted muscles.
4   Turn your hand back over and finish by pressing the side of each finger with your right thumb and finger from the top to the base, then gently pull each one. Repeat on the other hand.

MINI INDIAN-TYPE HEAD MASSAGE

This invigorating head massage complements the temple and neck sequence on pages 100-101. Working on your scalp in this way at lunchtime releases any taut muscles, improves your concentration, induces a feeling of wellbeing and gets any sluggish energy moving again.

Our heads are our power centres, where our brain organizes our busy days. It is not surprising, then, that they suffer from anxiety, emotional tension or headaches. Finger massaging around the crown of the head is very therapeutic, it recharges your energy levels, activates the lymphatic system to clear out toxins and soothes your tired spirit.

Massage your head (no oil is needed) for 5-10 minutes. Concentrate on easing any tight or knotted scalp areas.

1   With your forefinger and middle finger of one hand massage your scalp in a circular movement, slightly lifting your hair as you do so. This invigorates your scalp and revives flagging energies.
2   Using both hands, make circular movements with your fingertips all around your scalp. Grasp small handfuls of hair and give them a tug for instant tension relief.
3   Run your fingers over your face and then push them through your hair savouring the immediate energy surge and mental release. Repeat the process from the nape of your neck up to your crown, reducing any neck stiffness from your morning's concentrated work.

MID-AFTERNOON BOOSTERS

AT THIS TIME OF DAY YOUR ENERGY LEVELS REALLY START TO FLAG AND YOU NEED TO RE-ENERGIZE TO GET THROUGH THE REMAINDER OF THE AFTERNOON.

Mid-afternoon is when your energy levels can start to take a real dip, especially if the frustrations of the day are catching up with you. You may be feeling tense, have a slight headache or finding that some of your muscles are starting to ache. Try to stay upbeat, though, and let go of the day's anxieties. Don't dwell on any negative outcomes but focus on your successes.

Use the holistic energizers in this section to release the strains of the day and give you that last energy surge to keep you going for the rest of the afternoon.

Try to set aside a time to do a short energizer that recharges your physical state and emotional mood. By releasing any stress or rebalancing your inner energies, you can face the final responsibilities of the day with a lighter heart and renewed vigour.

EASING TENSION

As your working day continues you may find that your eyes become dry, tired and gritty from reading, driving or sitting in front of a computer for long periods. Bad lighting and air conditioning can also aggravate the problem making your eyes feel very dry and sore. Your neck muscles may also be starting to feel painful as they 'lock' and stiffen from constantly leaning forwards or staying too long in one position.

Taking time out briefly to ease the strain that has accumulated in your eye and neck muscles will give you that necessary energy surge to finish your day.

EXERCISE TIPS

Blink constantly for about 15 seconds to moisten dry eyes.

To perk up tired eyes, splash them alternately with hot and cold water for a few minutes.

PALMING

Covering your eyes so that they are in complete darkness can clear your head and refresh your eyes (see also pages 100-101).

1   Either sit with your elbows supported on a desk or table, or sit upright with your elbows on your chest, and cup your hands over your eyes. If you are at home, you can lie down to do this, but keep your knees bent.
2   Rub your palms together until they feel warm and then gently place your cupped hands over your closed eyes but do not touch them.
3   Breathe deeply as you enjoy the complete darkness, letting your mind empty as the warmth of your hands soothes your tired eyes. Breathe in stimulating energy into your eyes and breathe out any strain. Maintain your breathing rhythm for 5-10 minutes.

NECK ROLLS

Gently rub your tense neck muscles, then spend about 5 minutes doing these neck rolls to relax and loosen up any rigid muscles.

1   Stand or sit upright in a chair keeping your spine straight. Keep your shoulders down as you lean your head towards the right. Hold for 30 seconds, feeling the stretch in your neck and left shoulder. Relax your head, bring it back to the centre and repeat on the left side. Repeat several times on each side.

2   Drop your chin slowly down towards your chest and feel the stretch in the back of your neck; hold for 30 seconds then gently release. Repeat several times.

3   Take your right hand and put it on the back of your head. Push forwards gently with your hand to get an increased stretch in your neck; hold for 30 seconds then release. Repeat several times.

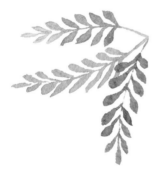

EXERCISE TIP

Always make sure that your shoulders do not round or stoop during these exercises as this posture can pull rather than relax the neck muscles. Try shrugging your shoulders to relax them first: squeeze your shoulders up towards your ears and then push them down as far as you can into your body. Repeat this sequence a few times and you'll feel tension simply disappear.

A TEA TONIC

The middle of the afternoon, particularly around 3–4p.m., is when energy levels slump and sometimes it can be hard to continue. Sipping a cup of herbal tea can act as a tonic (see also pages 32–33, 46 and 58), cleansing the blood and revitalizing the body organs. Some herbs, such as ginseng, are 'adaptogens' that fight or adapt to whatever problem the body is experiencing: if you are feeling tired, it will energize you; if you feel stressed it will calm you. If you are unable to buy ginseng powder, use a herbal tea bag instead. (Please note: you should avoid Korean ginseng if you are pregnant or have high blood pressure.)

GREEN TEA

There are many health benefits of drinking green tea, which is readily available in tea bags. As well as boosting the immune system, it contains powerful antioxidants that slow ageing and destroy free radicals (harmful reactive molecules that can damage body cells), thereby reducing the risk of cancer and heart disease.

GINSENG AND HONEY TEA

Ginseng makes a potent revitalizing tea that reduces physical or emotional stress. It can normalize blood sugar levels and stimulates the functioning of the brain and nervous system, aiding mental clarity.

Ingredients

3 teaspoons Korean ginseng powder (available from health stores or herbal shops)

1 cup of boiling water

1-2 teaspoons honey (optional)

Making the tea

1 Dissolve the ginseng powder in the boiling water and leave it to stand for 10 minutes.

2 Ginseng has a pleasant flavour of its own but some people prefer to add honey.

CRYSTAL POWER

Crystals are wonderful aids to healing as discussed on pages 34–35 and page 83. The vibrational frequencies they emit can bring your body and spirit back into balance. Natural quartz is one of the most versatile crystals. In a practical capacity its silicon chips are adapted for use in everyday commercial life to receive, store, amplify and transmit data in computers and in credit and smart cards. In healing, the crystal's ability to amplify energy, can harmonize all the *chakras* (see page 14), particularly the Crown chakra – your spiritual centre.

Use this natural quartz crystal in the middle of the afternoon to restore depleted energy and aid your mental awareness.

FENG SHUI TIP

Place your crystal in the northeast corner of your desk or study to stimulate your education and knowledge – your learning space.

CRYSTAL HEALING FOR ENERGY REBALANCING

Hold a cleansed crystal (see page 34) for 5-10 minutes to boost your chakras and to give you spiritual inspiration.

1   Sit comfortably in a chair holding your crystal next to your Solar plexus chakra (just below the breastbone). Close your eyes and tune in to the crystal's power, having already set its main intent (see page 34). Ask for increased energy flow through your *chakras*.

2   Now, place the crystal briefly on your Crown chakra on the top of your head and then your Third eye chakra in the middle of your forehead. Ask for spiritual and intuitive insight into current problems. Open your eyes and thank the crystal for its help.

CENTERING

The middle of the afternoon is a time when you can feel lethargic and a bit low, weighed down by the events and aggravations of the day. Spend a few minutes breathing out negative emotions that have accumulated inside to soothe you mind and spirit. This exercise can evoke a sense of calm as you realign your body's energies, smoothing out the flow of energy. Physically your heart and lungs will also benefit as they receive extra health-giving oxygen.By the end of this exercise your whole mind and body will feel energized and ready to cope with any challenging events that confront you later on in the afternoon.

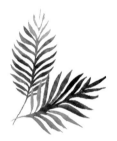

BREATHING TO REBALANCE

Practise this breathing exercise for about 5-10 minutes until you feel all irritations leaving you.

1   Sit comfortably in a chair, close your eyes and start taking slow, deep breaths from your diaphragm. When you have a regular breathing rhythm start to imagine that you are going down a well into the centre of your being.

2   As you inhale, take in the warm healing energy that is at the bottom of the well. As you breathe out, let go of all the negative thoughts and emotions that have built up during the day.

3   As you go deeper inside yourself, appreciate the silence, peace and self-love – no arguments, criticisms, fears or doubts can reach you here. Experience the bliss of connecting with your inner spirit in every part of your body. Slowly return up the well and come to, refreshed and ready for the rest of the afternoon's challenges.

ACHIEVING YOUR AIMS

Positive affirmations can help you achieve what you want, but you have got to believe they are going to happen. If you undertook the other affirmations earlier in the day (see pages 47 and 59) you will have benefited from the strength and confidence they have given you.

This afternoon affirmation can work on your goals later in the day or even the next morning. You may have an important meeting before you go home that is crucial to a current project so focus on a favourable outcome. Or you may have an appointment with your child's headteacher about his poor school-work performance, so use a phrase that shows the situation being mutually resolved.

ENERGY TIP

Smell some rosemary essential oil from a tissue (see page 56) as you do your affirmation to help increase your concentration.

AFTERNOON AFFIRMATION

Choose your positive phrase carefully, and make it short and to the point. Write it on a Post-it and stick it somewhere you can see it.

1   Sit comfortably, or walk up and down, as you repeat your phrase (out loud, preferably). In connection with the examples right, it may be: 'I am getting the extra staff I need for my project' or 'The headteacher offers a helpful strategy to improve my child's school performance'.
2   Really feel and mean what you are saying. Repeat 10–20 times to fix it in your subconscious and say it regularly throughout the afternoon.

CLEARING OUT

A work space, in an office, at home or any environment, needs to be well ordered, tidy and have good storage facilities for a good energy flow that encourages clear decision-making, creativity and business success. In feng shui, the art of furniture placement and energy flow, *chi* (energy) moves in spirals around a room. When this flow is obstructed by junk on the floor or surfaces, it becomes sluggish, slow and sticky affecting the atmosphere of your work area, so that you lack direction or enthusiasm for your projects.

Clearing out unwanted rubbish or clutter in mid-afternoon spurts over a week will create a substantial energy shift that allows space for new people or new projects to enter. Furthermore, it helps you to work with more confidence and drive.

CLUTTER TIP

The definition of work clutter is:

Something no longer needed or wanted.

A broken item or one that can't be fixed.

Something disliked or outmoded.

CLEVER STORAGE

If you have had a big clear-out but still have essential items that need to find 'homes', see where you could add new storage units; slim ones can fit in small spaces. Could you build more shelves above or below existing ones or fit more under sloping ceilings? Keep an eye out for clever storage items that can do more than one thing: space-saving shelves or tables that open up and store books or magazines hidden inside. Buy insert trays for slim metal cabinets that can sit under tables or desks to hold small pieces of stationery, home crafts, samples or other business items.

CLEARING YOUR WORK SPACE

Write a list of your worst clutter piles and start on them first. Spend 10-15 minutes clearing every day until the piles are gone.

1 Make the floor area a priority. Recycle any unwanted papers, magazines (file any clippings of interest) or outdated stationery. Go through boxes of old materials and be ruthless, keeping only what you use. In terms of storage, try to set up files on shelves to keep the floor free. Clear box files and, again, arrange them on shelves. Store anything that's not current in a cabinet or cupboard.

2 Empty wastepaper bins daily – they are pools of stagnancy.

3 Go through filing cabinets and thin house or work files down; save what is current, remove anything that is redundant and recycle what's not needed.

4 Clear your desk space. Keep invoices or bills in a bring-forward file or a pending tray. Refer on files or reports or store them in a cabinet as soon as you have dealt with them. Remove old Post-its and business cards, transferring phone numbers or useful information to your personal organizer or notebook. Deal with correspondence immediately, then file. Throw out broken pens, pencils, rulers and other old stationery, store essentials in a holder on the desk. Aim to leave your desk completely clear at the end of the day.

5 Sort through your bookshelves. Give away any duplicate books and any books that are no longer used. Save only up-to-date reference books and arrange logically on shelves; ditch any old ones as they keep you stuck in the past.

**WRITE A LIST
OF YOUR WORST
CLUTTER PILES AND
START ON THEM
FIRST.**

CLEAR YOUR COMPUTER

You're probably feeling renewed after clearing your work space (see pages 94–95), now it's time to sort out your computer. When both the hard disk and RAM are overloaded your computer becomes slow and inefficient. Conflicts between different software programs can also cause frustration, such as the computer 'freezing' or 'crashing'. When your computer is full and taking a long time to carry out simple commands, it can negatively affect you mentally and emotionally; the result is that you feel frustrated and out of control with your projects.

Try to spend 10 minutes or so each afternoon to clear out unwanted files, programs and correspondence. Have a plan of attack; how are you going to sort through all your various folders? Even after a day or two, you'll notice how your spirits rise as extraneous work disappears.

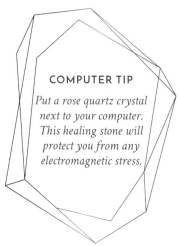

COMPUTER TIP

Put a rose quartz crystal next to your computer. This healing stone will protect you from any electromagnetic stress.

MAKING COMPUTER SPACE

Spend 10-15 minutes daily freeing up space on your computer so that you reduce any confusion in finding what you want. After a while, you may find you become almost obsessive about any unfiled items and you'll be delighted to see how organized your hard disk has become.

1   Go through your email inbox and delete any old messages. Print out or file onto the hard disk the ones you have to keep for reference. Remember to delete any sent mail as well.

2   Look through your hard disk and delete or archive onto storage disks correspondence files or projects that are no longer current. Remove software programs that are out of date (or get some professional help if you are unsure) or redundant.

PURIFYING A WORK SPACE

After your clear-out, you may be left with a slight,
musty atmosphere as old dusty articles have been
shifted from the floor and surfaces. Once you have
cleaned everywhere thoroughly, spend a short
time space clearing the room or desk to dispel any
lingering stagnancy. The technique can cleanse the
existing *chi*, leaving a new bright, vibrancy that will
encourage a positive working attitude.

There are several methods of space clearing (see
pages 116–123) but if you work in an open-plan
space (where other people are involved), the
simplest is misting essential oils.

SPACE CLEARING YOUR WORK AREA

Spend a few minutes spraying aromatic essential oils
around your work area to change the atmosphere
and boost productivity.

1 Put 4 drops of oil in a mister bottle and half fill
with water; mix (see also page 117). Spray around
you first to revitalize your aura (see also page 131).
2 If you have a contained work space, spray round
it in a clockwise direction, misting high into the
corners, asking for a more positive, successful and
creative space. Also mist round and under your
desk and over your computer and chair.

**STIMULATING AND
CLEANSING OILS**

*Use eucalyptus,
lemongrass or rosemary
essential oils.*

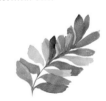

COLOUR HEALING

As your energy levels plummet mid-afternoon, try this colour exercise to boost your body organs and glands and your *chakras* (see page 14 and 49).

The healing colour vibrations that enter our bodies and *chakras* (see page 14) through sunlight are necessary for them to function well. Spending so much time indoors, working or doing chores at home, can mean we don't always get a natural 'top up' of this sunlight energy, which later in the day can leave us feeling a bit drained and lacking in motivation. Visualize the seven colours entering your body and flooding it with colour to rebalance your energy.

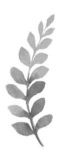

COLOUR VISUALIZATION

Spend 5-10 minutes regularly filling your body with the healing colours of the rainbow.

1 Sit comfortably and take some deep breaths from your diaphragm. Now visualize a bright red colour coming up your legs into your Root chakra (lower pelvis); feel it dispelling your fears.

2 Now, change the colour to a rich orange and see it filling your Sacral chakra (lower abdomen) and bringing joy. Next, see the colour as a bright yellow flooding your Solar plexus chakra (upper abdomen) and clearing your mind and emotions.

3 As the yellow fades, bring in a loving, purifying green colour to your Heart chakra (over the heart). Then visualize a turquoise in your Throat chakra (upper chest and throat) and sense how it helps your self-expression.

4 Let the blue fade to a deep indigo that washes over your Third eye chakra (middle of your forehead) and boosts your intuitive powers. Finally, see a soft violet colour entering your Crown chakra (top of your head), stimulating your spirit (your 'higher self'). As the colour disappears, come to, feeling revitalized and recharged.

DOWSING FOR COLOUR

If you lack energy but don't quite know what chakra or which body area body is suffering, find out the colour you currently lack by using the dowsing technique.

Dowsing is an ancient technique that utilizes divining rods or pendulums to detect the presence of substances such as water and oil or unnatural earth energies. The technique works by asking questions of your subconscious mind (your inner self). Responses come through the electromagnetic energies emitted by your hands. This method also works on your body, so you can easily check which chakra is not balanced or underfunctioning.

THE DOWSING TECHNIQUE

Spend a few minutes daily dowsing to find out which colour (sometimes more than one) your body is lacking.

1 Hold your pendulum loosely in your hand and ask it which direction is 'yes'. It will spin either clockwise or anticlockwise. Ask it for 'no' and note these directions down. Finally ask for a 'don't know' response, which is normally swinging from side to side.
2 Now, hold the pendulum over each coloured card and ask in turn 'do I need this colour today'. Write down the responses. Keep the coloured card or cards you need in front of you, or with you, to look at regularly to absorb their healing vibrations.

ESSENTIAL EQUIPMENT

Buy a pendulum with a clear quartz crystal or make one by hanging a bead on a cord 15 cm (6 in) long.

Make seven small cards of the chakra colours in red, orange, yellow, green, turquoise, indigo, violet.

MASSAGE RELIEF

Massaging your head mid-afternoon with simple hand movements is a wonderful release for any mental or emotional stress that has developed. It can also remove the strain from taut muscles and prevent the onset of a painful and debilitating headache (see page 57).

MASSAGING YOUR HEAD IS A WONDERFUL RELEASE FOR ANY MENTAL OR EMOTIONAL STRESS.

When your body is under stress, blood flow becomes restricted through the veins and arteries creating that 'tight' uncomfortable feeling, particularly in areas such as the head. As adrenaline is released from the adrenal glands to help you cope with a situation where quick reactions are needed, your heart beats faster and your muscles begin to ache as they tense or 'harden'. Working long hours hunched over a desk or driving for too long in a rigid position can also cause a stiff neck and eye strain.

MIND AND BODY RELEASE

Research by an Austrian psychoanalyst called Wilhelm Reich in the mid-twentieth century first reinforced massage as a holistic therapy. He expressed the belief that the mind and body were interconnected and that emotions such as anger or despair could be held in tense body areas and require release for good health and wellbeing.

HEAD MASSAGE TECHNIQUE

This easy routine takes only 5-10 minutes and requires no oils.
By applying pressure around your eyes and doing fingertip massage
around your temples and the back of your neck, you can improve
blood flow, release tension and encourage better oxygen flow to
create a sense of wellbeing.

1   Close your eyes. Intertwine your fingers and press your thumbs
    into the corners of your eyes. Hold for about 3 seconds and then
    repeat 6 times to reduce eye strain.

2   With your right forefinger and thumb pinch your nose at the
    top; left-handers may prefer to use their left hand. Hold for about
    3 seconds, release, then repeat 6 times to clear your vision and
    ease tiredness.

3   With you right forefinger, press on your Third eye chakra in the
    centre of your forehead. Hold for about 6 seconds, then release
    and repeat 4 times to shift any energy blockages.

4   With the first and second fingers of your right hand, push up from
    your eyebrows and over to the temple area to ease tension. Move
    across the face from right to left.

5   With your fingers apart, hold the back of your head and circle your
    thumbs around the fleshy area at the base of your skull to relieve
    neck muscle tension. Work around the area for a couple of minutes,
    stopping if it feels painful. Repeat once more.

6   Put your hands at the base of the back of your neck and move them
    up to your crown. Clutch a handful of hair each side and tug for a
    few seconds. Now slide your fingers to the temples at the side of
    your head, clutch your hair again and tug gently from side to side.
    Repeat both actions 2 or 3 times, then smooth your fingers through
    your hair and feel your mental frustrations lifting.

SOOTHING REFLEXOLOGY

The afternoon is often the time when the pace of a busy day catches up with you. If you have been on the phone constantly or typing important emails, or spent hours in meetings or rushing about organizing children you may well feel pressured. These short reflexology routines can give you instant benefits and reduce unpleasant stress symptoms.

Reflexology (see pages 64–65) is a massage technique that works on pressure points on the hands and feet to increase energy flow in the ten 'reflex' zones and to remove any existing blockages in the muscles and organs that may be causing pain. The two routines here work mainly on the hands and help smooth out energy blocks to reduce the gripes of a stressed stomach and the twinges and soreness of early repetitive strain injury (RSI) symptoms in your fingers, hands, wrists and shoulders.

REFLEXOLOGY TIPS

Wash your hands before and also after a treatment as you are working with stagnant energy.

Work gently on any sensitive areas with the tips of your middle finger and forefinger.

THESE SHORT
REFLEXOLOGY
ROUTINES
CAN GIVE YOU
INSTANT BENEFITS
AND REDUCE
UNPLEASANT
STRESS SYMPTOMS.

———

RELIEF FOR A STRESSED STOMACH

Work on the points for several minutes if your stomach is reacting badly to a stressful day.

1 Press with your left thumb on the liver point of your right hand, halfway down from your little finger. Also work on the gallbladder point, in and down from your second finger.
2 If you have cramping stomach pains, work on the thyroid point on the outside of your right hand in between your thumb and your forefinger.
3 Also work on the parathyroid reflexes between your thumb and your forefinger and the solar plexus point in the middle of your hand under the third finger. Stimulate the diaphragm point, too, which curves across the middle of the hand from under the little finger.

RELEASING RSI-TYPE SYMPTOMS

Press on these points for several minutes to ease strain in your hands, arms and shoulders.

1 Start working with your thumbs across the top of the sole of one foot, concentrating on the neck (under the big toe) and shoulder girdle (under the little toe). Do the same on the other foot. Then work on the arm and hand reflexes down the top half of your right foot from your little toe. Alternatively work on your hands.
2 Work on the hip and leg reflexes further down the side of the right foot to move energy down the body. Finally stretch and rotate each finger of both hands to break the stress-holding patterns.

LETTING GO OF TENSION

As the evening draws near, you can become aware of many tense areas in your muscles from the rigours of the day. Recognizing where they are, and how they have become tense, is the first step towards loosening or relaxing them, and preventing it happening again. When you release muscle tension you can also relieve a headache or backache that has built up during the day. The process also benefits and helps clear your mind as it automatically quietens as you focus on letting go.

Once you know the muscle-releasing technique well, you will sense when your muscles are tightening and be easily able to relax them.

WHEN YOU RELEASE MUSCLE TENSION YOU CAN ALSO RELIEVE A HEADACHE OR BACKACHE.

QUICK RELAXATION ROUTINE

If you have an important meeting or want to unwind before going out and your muscles feel very taut, carry out this 2-3-minute routine, to release any tension.

1   Concentrate on breathing slowly and choose a cue word such as 'release' and repeat it in your mind as you start to relax.
2   Take a deep breath and at the same time clench a group of muscles in areas of your body where tension gathers, such as your face, neck, shoulders, chest and stomach.
3   As you breathe out, let go of your muscles, feeling all the tightness and tension simply slipping away.

THE MUSCLE-RELEASING TECHNIQUE

Work with this technique for at least 10 minutes, maybe more, to loosen up your body and inspire your mind.

1 Sit comfortably or lie down. Close your eyes or focus on a fixed point ahead of you. Take 4 long, deep breaths from your diaphragm, and then breathe with a light, even rhythm.

2 Now take your attention to your toes, breathe in and tense them for about 5 seconds, then let go as you breathe out, feeling all the tightness flowing out. Notice what effect it has on your whole body. Repeat once or twice, then move on to your lower legs and repeat the movement there, again seeing how it feels in the rest of your body.

3 In the same way, work up your body tensing and releasing the major muscle groups in turn: your thighs, buttocks, lower back, stomach, chest, shoulders, arms, hands and neck, noticing any tense or tight areas loosening up.

4 When you get to your face, screw it up tightly, hold for 5 seconds and release. Then open your eyes and mouth wide, again holding for 5 seconds before releasing. Repeat twice.

5 Now tense your whole body from your toes to your head, hold for a few seconds and let go: see how heavy and loose your body feels when you let go. Relax for a few moments, and then open your eyes, feeling recharged and ready to continue your afternoon.

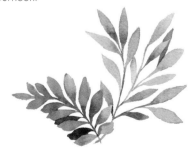

EVENING REFRESHERS

SIT DOWN AND REFLECT ON YOUR DAY; SOME ARE BEST FORGOTTEN, BUT FOR MOST DAYS YOU CAN LOOK BACK ON YOUR ACHIEVEMENTS WITH SATISFACTION.

When you reach the end of a busy day, you can feel quite drained, mentally and emotionally. What is more, if you have a long journey home from work or need to put your children to bed before you can wind down, you can feel even more exhausted when you finally get some time to yourself. Sit down and reflect on your day; some are best forgotten, but for most days you can look back on your achievements with satisfaction. Give yourself some well-deserved praise for everything that you have done.

Now you have started to relax, choose an exercise from this section to harmonize your inner and outer chi. Lift your spirits with a wonderful scented bath, dismiss the cares of the day by dancing to some lively music, do some drumming to raise the energy levels in your living room or ease the aches of the day with a neck and shoulder massage with oils.

Select the evening energizer that you know will work best for how you feel and will give you optimism and verve for the hours ahead.

CANDELIGHT BATHING

Letting go of the physical and mental tensions of a busy day coping with children, dealing with customers or spending hours in front of a computer is essential to your wellbeing. If you work outside the home, you also have the added aggravation of commuting. One of the best ways of freeing all the day's stresses, and restoring your energy for the evening ahead, is to spend some time on your own soaking in a perfumed bath.

Essential oils (see page 30–31 and 56–57) evoke the wonderful scents of the plants or flowers from which they are extracted. When they are added to a warm bath their therapeutic aromas are breathed in and are also absorbed by your skin, producing immediate psychological and physical benefits that will last all evening.

OIL TIP

Maximize your benefits by making a blend of oils for massaging into your skin. Mix 3 drops of each chosen oil into 20 ml/4 teaspoons of sweet almond or grapeseed base oil. After your bath, rub the oil well into your skin, starting at your feet and working upwards towards the heart.

INSPIRING CANDLES

Soft, flickering candles around the bath or in wall sconces can create a soft, relaxing ambience when you are soaking the day away. They can also lift the energy flow in a bathroom, which is naturally sluggish and yin (passive). This is because candles link to the Fire element in feng shui and are considered yang (positive). You can also bring in some colour therapy by using green candles to harmonize your energy; white candles can bring protection.

**ONE OF THE BEST
WAYS OF FREEING
ALL THE DAY'S
STRESSES IS TO
SPEND SOME TIME
ON YOUR OWN
SOAKING IN A
PERFUMED BATH.**

FRAGRANT BATH WITH MAGICAL CANDLES

Choose an essential oil blend (right) or experiment with mixing your own to find the one that calms your soul and lifts your spirits. (Safe note: always remember to extinguish all candles after finishing your bath.)

1   Run a bath. When it is full put 3-4 drops each of your chosen oil blend in the water and agitate gently to mix them in.
2   Sink into the bath, close your eyes and let the oils do their work. Shut down your mind and feel all the aches of the day dissolving into the water. Stay in the bath for at least 15 minutes to absorb the curative qualities of the oils.

HEALING OILS

Lavender and basil oil to calm emotions and clear the mind.

Geranium and jasmine oil to ease nervous tension and lift the mood.

Lime and ylang ylang oil to reduce any anxiety and stimulate sluggish organs.

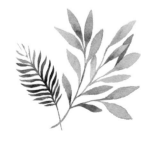

SOOTHE AND STRETCH

Neck and shoulder tension often builds up over a working day. Being rigid in the same position for a long time is a common trigger. When muscles are tight they feel sore and uncomfortable, and the veins and arteries become restricted, resulting in poor blood flow.

The lymphatic system can also become sluggish and does not pick up toxins so easily. Knotted muscles are also thought to restrict the flow of *chi* (see page 9) around the body and can affect your mental and emotional outlook.

A SOOTHING OIL MIXTURE

Mix 3 drops each of lavender and geranium essential oil into 20 ml/ 4 teaspoons sweet almond or grapeseed base oil.

NECK AND SHOULDER MASSAGE

Massaging taut muscles eases the tension, releases endorphins (the 'happy hormones') into the body, increases blood flow to the organs and slows your breathing. Knead a soothing oil mixture into your shoulder and neck muscles for about 5-10 minutes to remove daily strains.

1 Remove your top or slip it over your shoulders. Sit in a chair and rub oil into your hands. With your right hand, work on your left shoulder, kneading the muscles to loosen the tension. Move up and down the shoulder several times. Then, repeat on your right shoulder using your left hand.

2 With both hands, use your fingers to squeeze and release the neck muscles, working from the bottom of your neck up to the base of the skull and down again. Repeat several times. Finally, with your right hand only, knead or grip your neck muscles, several times until any tightness relaxes.

NECK AND SHOULDER STRETCHING

If you return home from work with a knotted neck and stiff shoulders but have insufficient time to do the neck and shoulder massage opposite, try this quick routine.

It is a simple stretching exercise using a rolled bath towel that can alleviate the tension in your aching muscles in just a few minutes, leaving you rejuvenated for the evening ahead.

You can get your blood circulation flowing more smoothly by stretching your neck and shoulders muscles with a bath towel in this simple routine.

1 Kneel on a mat on the floor in your bedroom or bathroom. Roll up a warm bath towel and put it round your neck, holding it with both hands. Lean back and arch your neck and hold for a few seconds, then release, feeling the tension lessening. Repeat 6 times.

2 Pull the ends of the towel down and wrap around your shoulders. Holding the towel tightly, push your fists into the small of your back, moving your elbows back to increase the pressure on your tight shoulders, and open your chest. Hold for a few seconds then release, feeling tension knots dissolving as you do so. Repeat 6 times.

ENERGY TIP

As you are stretching your upper body, repeat this relaxing mantra out loud 10 times: 'I am releasing all stress and tension from my neck'

POWERFUL BREATHING

This type of breathing is a form of pranayama (breath control) that is used in yoga (see page 17). Practising this technique, where you breathe in through the left nostril and then the right, encourages the breath to flow smoothly through the seven main chakras in the body (see page 14) and remove any negative energy blockages that it encounters. It balances the body's masculine (the right nostril) and feminine (the left nostril) energies that need to be in harmony for complete wellbeing. This powerful breathing technique also helps to purify the nervous system, clear the mind and relax the body. It is often used before meditation.

Practise this in the early evening to clear the worries and anxieties of the day and leave you refreshed to enjoy the rest of the night.

MINI MEDITATION

Do this short meditation for about 5 minutes at the end of your working day to quieten a busy mind.

1 Sit cross-legged on the floor and follow the meditation technique on page 41. As you focus on one thought try to let go of the day. As work thoughts or problems intrude let them float past you and visualize them flying out of a nearby window.
2 As your mind stills and you start to relax, feel a sense of peace filling your body and mind. Just before you open your eyes, praise yourself for what you have achieved during the day, don't focus on any negatives, instead just send good energy towards the following day.

ALTERNATE NOSTRIL BREATHING

Use this method to breathe for a few minutes. You will notice that the breath is stronger and louder on the right.

1   Sit cross-legged on the floor or in the lotus or half-lotus position with your spine straight. Put your arms on your knees. Touch your first finger and thumb together of your left hand and fold in the middle three fingers of your right hand, keeping your thumb and little finger extended. These gestures are hand mudras, which are subtle movements that embody a spiritual meaning. Breathe deeply and evenly from the diaphragm.

2   Lift up your right hand and block your left nostril with your little finger. Breathe in and then out deeply through the right nostril letting all the air out of your lungs. Repeat this breathing process for 10 breaths.

3   Now block the right nostril with your right thumb and breathe in and out for about 10 seconds. Repeat the exercises 3–5 times on each side, and then finish by breathing deeply through both nostrils again as in the first step.

PRACTISING THIS TECHNIQUE ENCOURAGES THE BREATH TO FLOW SMOOTHLY THROUGH THE SEVEN MAIN CHAKRAS IN THE BODY AND REMOVE ANY NEGATIVE ENERGY BLOCKAGES THAT IT ENCOUNTERS.

———

EXPRESSIVE DANCING

Dance movement is an arts therapy that shows how a person expresses any emotional disturbance through their body movements. Everyone has an individual way of moving; in a class a therapist analyses each person working out their strengths and sees where they may benefit from developing more self-awareness and group interaction.

YOU CAN DANCE AT HOME IN THE EARLY EVENING TO RELEASE ANY EMOTIONAL UPSET AND ANGST FROM THE DAY.

In a simpler way you can use the dance technique at home in the early evening to release any emotional upset and angst from the day. Dancing can also increase your energy levels as you enthusiastically move all your limbs, shaking out all held tension. Music evokes powerful emotions in everyone: classical pieces can uplift our spirits, soothe our souls or even make us cry, while popular music can make us shout with joy as we sing along to a favourite number.

Regularly dancing to stimulating music with a strong beat, such as rock, jazz or Latin music, such as salsa, can give your body and mind a welcome release and some escapism after a busy, demanding or upsetting day.

DANCE CLASSES

If you really enjoy dancing, consider joining a weekly dance class locally, such as Ceroc or Le Roc (jiving techniques) or salsa. Classes are available in many areas and can be very sociable. They normally start with lessons in the early part of the evening with a 'freestyle' section later, where everyone has the opportunity to dance with each other.

DANCE AWAY FRUSTRATIONS

Create your own special space to dance away your daily frustrations for about 10 minutes each night. It can help remove energy blocks and give you the mental stimulation to enjoy the evening ahead.

1   Prepare the room in which you are going to dance. Make sure it is warm, dim the lights, close the curtains, turn off the phone so you are not disturbed. Wear some loose and comfortable clothing and choose a lively dance track.

2   Turn the volume up to a reasonable level and start to dance, building up from a slow rhythm to something faster and more energetic. If there are lyrics you love, express yourself further by singing along with them (see page 81).

3   It may feel strange to start with, but don't worry if you are not used to dancing by yourself - no one can see you. Get into the rhythm of the music, feel the beat moving through your legs, hips, shoulders and arms. Start to dance faster, doing more energetic movements and feel how your muscles become less stiff and move with more fluidity. Dance for about 10 minutes or more until you lose the worries of the day and feel new energy freely surging through your body.

ROOM PURIFYING

Hoarding junk in your home can block its positive energy flow, while arguments, upsets, illness and other incidents all leave their energetic imprint on the building. By removing clutter and using a purifying technique you can raise the energy frequency, creating balance and harmony once more.

At the end of a long day the atmosphere in certain rooms of your home can often seem a bit sluggish or dull. If this is left unchanged, you can start to feel lethargic and uninspired about the evening ahead. Try these easy, refreshing techniques to lift the flagging energy levels and clear out negative energy. You'll feel instantly better, and able to look forward to a great night out or a creative evening at home.

ENERGY TIP

If you don't have essential oils, spray rooms with spring water for a quick energy uplift and a healthy negative-ion rich environment (a feeling similar to being by the sea).

CLAPPING

Clapping is a wonderful, simple sound technique that gets rid of any stagnant or low energy areas in a room by loosening the energetic imprint. Clap for 5–10 minutes, first practising a few fast claps in a corner. If they sound muffled or very dull, the chi (energy) is very low and you will need to clap from floor to ceiling to disperse it.

1   Stand in the doorway of your room and focus on clearing dead energy as you clap clockwise round the room, doing small, fast claps in corners to see if the energy is depleted. Do louder, larger claps when the energy sounds muffled or dull and needs extra clearing.
2   When the dead energy has lifted, your claps will sound sharp and clear. Clap round each room that needs cleansing, until all the negativity has dispersed.
3   After about 10 minutes clapping, stand still in the room and sense the brighter, clearer energy. The changed and revived atmosphere feels similar to when you have opened all the windows to let in fresh air.

SPACE CLEARING WITH OILS

Essential oils stimulate the olfactory nerves in our nostrils, producing an immediate mood change. Many different oils are available (see page 31), and when heated in vaporizers or added to baths, they stimulate or calm the senses. By misting oils into a room's atmosphere you can immediately produce a vibrant and uplifting or calm and relaxed atmosphere, depending on the oil used. You are also left with a wonderful residual fragrance.

1   Fill a mister bottle (ideally made of glass, as it keeps better) with water and mix in about 5-6 drops of your chosen oil.

2   Starting at the door, spray your aura first (see page 131) and concentrate on your personal energy clearing. Then mist the scent into the atmosphere as you walk clockwise around the rooms that need purifying for about 10 minutes, spraying more of the oil mist into any dark, unused corners.

3   Stand back and sense how the energy in the room has changed for the better. For a serious uplift, repeat daily for a week.

USEFUL OILS

For an invigorating, refreshing ambience try tangy oils such as mandarin, lime, grapefruit or lemon.

To calm use lavender, geranium, camomile or frankincense.

For a deep cleansing of stale energy juniper, clary sage or pine oils are best. (See also page 31 for oils and their effects.)

RHYTHMIC DRUMMING

Drumming is another sound technique that can change the atmosphere in a room in your home for the better, especially if an upset has occurred there the previous evening. The drum's powerful rhythm and vibrations can immediately create a substantial energetic shift in a room, improving the flow of *chi* and the overall atmosphere.

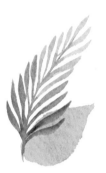

Many Native American Indian tribes used drums, believing that the drumbeat represented the heart of Mother Earth and that drums carried the life spirit. Modern shamans still use the drum to get them in a trance-like state for 'journeying' (a technique similar to visualization) to seek advice from spirit guides. The hypnotic beat actually affects their brain waves putting them in a state of altered consciousness.

DRUMMING TIPS

If you do not want to buy your own drum, choose a shamanic drumming CD (available from alternative shops) and play it quite loud to clear your chosen room.

1 Drumming is a very absorbing practice, if you drum in the early evening you may find you lose yourself in its hypnotic rhythm and forget all your cares and worries.
2 Drumming is particularly effective in clearing emotional energy, when there have been tears or an angry outburst, for example.
3 Drumming is the best technique to use if you feel the energy in a room is very congested and uninviting.

DRUMMING TO INCREASE POSITIVITY

Hand-held circular-frame drums made from animal skin are the most common types used for space clearing but any type can be used. Drum for about 10 minutes or until you feel the energy in the room has changed.

1 Many drums are held between the knees when you are drumming, so if you buy this type sit in the middle of the room to drum. But, if you use a hand-held drum, walk clockwise around the room from the doorway.

2 Hold the drum quietly in your hands for a few minutes to connect to it. Start drumming with a two-beat rhythm, keeping your wrists loose. This is the beat you first heard in the womb: the lubb-dupp of your mother's heartbeat. Let your body relax and your breathing deepen. As you develop the rhythm and strengthen your connection with your drum, instinctively quicken or slow the beat when it seems right. You will naturally start to drum faster when you encounter some stagnant energy.

3 If you are sitting to drum, towards the end of your 10 minutes, stand up and go to drum in each corner of the room to lift sluggish energy there. When you have finished, thank your drum for its help in space clearing the room and store it in a safe place.

THE DRUM'S POWERFUL RHYTHM AND VIBRATIONS CAN IMMEDIATELY CREATE A SUBSTANTIAL ENERGETIC SHIFT IN A ROOM.

———

UPLIFTING TONING

Toning is a simple purifying technique where you use the power of your own voice to change the energy flow. Anyone can use this technique; you just need to be able to hold one note for an extended time. If you arrive home and feel the atmosphere is flat in your living room, go round the room toning for a short time and notice how quickly you bring the 'buzz' back into the space.

Before your start toning a room, you need to find your own unique sounds. So, relax your body, particularly your face and jaw, and practise with a vowel tone such as 'ahhhh' or a musical scale such as 'doh'. Say it louder and louder and see how it grows from inside your body and reverberates around the room.

AFTER TONING FOR A SHORT TIME YOU WILL NOTICE HOW QUICKLY YOU BRING THE 'BUZZ' BACK INTO THE SPACE.

PURIFYING A ROOM WITH TONING

Practise with your chosen tone until it is strong and clear. 'Tone' round the room for about 10 minutes until you feel a new vibrancy in its energy.

1 Start toning at the room's doorway. Walk clockwise around the room, increasing the volume as you walk round. Feel the sound you are making and the 'sound' of the room becoming one.
2 Walk round and round in circles, stopping and toning louder in any stagnant areas where you hear the tone changing and becoming more muffled.

USING A SINGING BOWL

A singing bowl is another potent sound instrument that quickly lifts dull energy in living areas in the early evening. It can also literally 'clear the air' and harmonize the vibrations if you have had people staying, or workmen in.

Authentic singing bowls come from Tibet or Nepal and are made of seven metals, one of which must be gold, silver or platinum. The round bowl represents a vessel that can receive good luck but which can also capture bad energy and transform it into good energy. Stroking the bowl with a mallet produces a wonderful humming, energy field that spirals out from the bowl and back into its centre, dispelling any stagnancies while also pulling in positive vibrations.

CHANGING ENERGY WITH A SINGING BOWL

Play your singing bowl for about 10 minutes to clear a room and see how vibrant the atmosphere becomes.

1   Sit in the middle of your room; your bowl needs to be stationary to reach full volume. Connect with your bowl, then place it on the flat palm of one hand and start stroking its outer or inner edge with its wooden mallet.

2   Move the mallet around your bowl firmly, feeling it start to 'sing'. Ask it to clear your inner energies as the beautiful sound whirls around you, purifying the room. Thank your bowl for its help and store wrapped in a silk scarf.

PURIFYING SMUDGING

One of the strongest ways of cleansing negativity from a room is smudging. It is well known for clearing predecessor energy when you move home and is particularly effective for cleansing a room after a bad argument or if someone has been ill. So use this purifier in the early evening if you feel a substantial change is needed in the energy levels of some of your rooms.

Smudging is an ancient Native American tradition that uses smoke from burning herbal sticks to purify a space. Smudge sticks, which are available from alternative health shops or via mail order, are commonly made from sage, sweetgrass and rosemary (see page 33) because of their strong purification powers, which have been known about since ancient times.

USE THIS PURIFIER IN THE EARLY EVENING IF YOU FEEL A SUBSTANTIAL CHANGE IS NEEDED IN THE ENERGY LEVELS OF SOME OF YOUR ROOMS.

Feathers are traditionally used to waft the smoke around the room when you are smudging, as they are believed to connect you to the spirit world. If you buy or find a feather to use, always honour it and the bird it came from, and store it in a special place. Some countries restrict taking any part of a bird from the wild, so check your local regulations before taking a feather from outside.

SMUDGING TO SHIFT NEGATIVITY

Smudge the healing smoke around the room for 5-10 minutes to remove any negative vibrations from the space. Use one sage smudge stick and a feather, if you have one, for this exercise.

1 Light your smudge stick and blow out the flame. Hold it over a flameproof dish to catch any embers. When it is smoking well, flick smoke with your hand or your feather all round your body to cleanse your aura (your body's spiritual energy field) of all the 'debris' you have picked up during the day.

2 Now, from the doorway of your room, walk round in a clockwise direction wafting the smoke with a flick of your wrist in front of you, make sure it reaches right into corners where energy tends to stagnate. Focus in your mind on cleansing the room of any specific problem.

3 If you feel any 'sticky' areas in the room where the energy seems different, spend a little longer there wafting the smoke around. When you have finished, put out your smudge stick in an ashtray or dowse it quickly with water under a running tap. Store in a cupboard for using again another time.

SMUDGING TIPS

When you light your smudge stick, let it burn for a few seconds before blowing out the flame so that it smoulders well, giving out a good smoke trail.

Open all the windows in a room to let the smoke out after smudging.

After smudging with a feather, shake it well to discharge its energy.

EVENING YOGA

At the end of a long day your body and mind can be in need of some rejuvenation to enjoy the evening ahead. Yoga (see pages 50–51) is a wonderful exercise discipline that can relieve both mental and physical stress. The moves encourage suppleness and promote better inner energy flow, bringing harmony to the mind, body and spirit.

These easy poses take only 5–10 minutes and help to release accumulated tension in the spine, calm the mind and clear your thoughts and emotions. The Child's pose releases any spinal tension while the knee twists that follow tone and realign the spine. Always wear loose, comfortable clothing for your yoga session (see page 51).

THE MOVES ENCOURAGE SUPPLENESS AND PROMOTE BETTER INNER ENERGY FLOW, BRINGING HARMONY TO THE MIND, BODY AND SPIRIT.

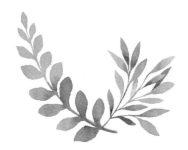

CHILD'S POSE

This exercise takes a few minutes and relieves all the spinal tension of the day, soothes your mind and nervous system, and alleviates any stiffness in the neck and shoulders.

1   Kneel on all fours on a mat on the floor. Put your arms out in front of you and breathe in, keeping your head in line with the rest of your spine.
2   Breathe out, pushing your hips all the way back so that you sit on your heels, your head looks at the floor, your arms go forward and your chest balances on your knees.
3   Move your arms behind you so that they hold your heels, as you breathe in and out deeply. Then move your hands further up your feet. Hold for a few minutes until you feel all your tension releasing. Repeat a few times if your back is very tense.

KNEE TWISTS

These twists can release any stress still held in your muscles and spine. They also relieve backache and boost the blood supply to the spinal discs and nerves.

1   Lie flat on the floor on your mat with your knees bent and your arms stretched out to the side, palms facing downwards. Make sure your neck and head are in line with your spine.
2   Breathe in and as you breathe out, start to take your knees down to the floor on your right in one fluid movement, letting your stomach muscles facilitate the twist. As your knees reach the floor, turn your head to the left. Only move your pelvis, do not twist your shoulders and chest as this can put strain on your back.
3   Breathe in and bring your knees back to the centre and hold briefly.
4   Now take your legs down to the left and turn your head to the right. Perform the exercise for several minutes or until you feel all your body tension has gone.

LATE-NIGHT CLEANSERS

LATE EVENING IS THE TIME FOR A MAJOR CLEANSE
OF YOUR MIND, BODY AND SPIRIT SO THAT YOU ARE
REVITALIZED FOR THE NEXT DAY.

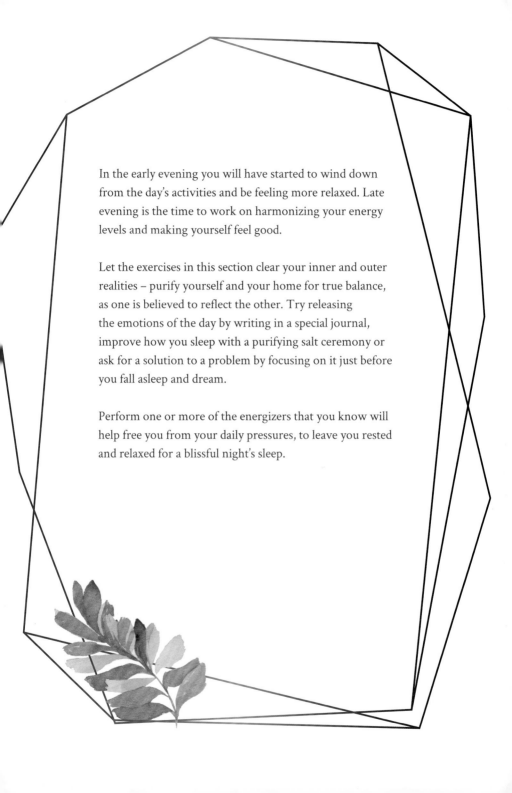

In the early evening you will have started to wind down from the day's activities and be feeling more relaxed. Late evening is the time to work on harmonizing your energy levels and making yourself feel good.

Let the exercises in this section clear your inner and outer realities – purify yourself and your home for true balance, as one is believed to reflect the other. Try releasing the emotions of the day by writing in a special journal, improve how you sleep with a purifying salt ceremony or ask for a solution to a problem by focusing on it just before you fall asleep and dream.

Perform one or more of the energizers that you know will help free you from your daily pressures, to leave you rested and relaxed for a blissful night's sleep.

INSIGHTFUL JOURNALLING

If you feel upset and raw after a turbulent day, 'journalling' is a positive way of writing down your feelings and emotions about what has happened. You can write whatever you like. Perhaps you are angry with a colleague or you are upset because your childcarer has let you down at short notice. Just let all your thoughts come out.

Journalling is a technique often used by life coaches to get people to connect with their inner selves and find their true path. Too often we are so busy with our external lives, we do not listen to our inner 'voices' or messages. These are our internal thoughts that link us to our future.

If you do some journalling on a daily basis it can help support you emotionally and give you insight to old problems and the bright new future you want to create.

'JOURNALLING' IS A POSITIVE WAY OF WRITING DOWN YOUR FEELINGS AND EMOTIONS

THE INNER CHILD

Part of our subconscious mind contains our 'inner child' – the part of us that stood still at about four or five years old. This inner child holds our fears and worries and longs to be loved. It also hangs on to childhood beliefs: so if you were told as a child 'You'll never be a success' or 'Earning money is a struggle', your inner child will still believe this, until, that is, it receives different instructions. Journalling gives you a chance to update and rewrite these beliefs.

JOURNALLING TO CLEAR THE DAY

Write down your daily 'ups and downs' in a special journal, or on your computer, to let go of any emotional upsets, and to seek guidance for any changes you need to make.

1   Sit comfortably at a table or at your computer. Close your eyes and take some deep breaths from your diaphragm. As your breathing slows stare ahead of you at a fixed point in the wall and quieten your busy mind.

2   When you are really relaxed, start writing in your journal or on your computer. Write what you are feeling inside, do not worry if it does not seem to make sense or you seem to be ranting. Don't let your ego question what you are doing, just let all your thoughts flow out; you will find a reason for them later.

3   If any old emotion or memory pops into your head as you are writing, put it down, everything comes out for a reason. After about 10 minutes or when you have covered three or four sides of your journal (if writing) stop writing. Sit still for a moment to recover from your emotional release and to disconnect from your subconscious mind before continuing your evening.

CRYSTAL HEALING

Crystals are powerful healers as they can harmonize any existing distortions in the rhythms of our bodies and chakras (see also pages 34–35, 83 and 91). Amethyst is one of the best healing stones to use as it has the ability to absorb the negativity of the day, and can also calm and purify the body and spirit. Furthermore, it can draw out any anger, fears or resentment that have built up in the body.

Use a piece of amethyst in the late evening to physically and psychically cleanse you, so that you are ready to enjoy a calm and peaceful night's sleep.

USE A PIECE OF AMETHYST IN THE LATE EVENING TO PHYSICALLY AND PSYCHICALLY CLEANSE YOU.

CRYSTAL CEREMONY FOR MIND AND BODY

Hold a cleansed amethyst crystal (see page 34) for about 10 minutes in your lap and then hold briefly to your Third eye chakra (the middle of your forehead) and your Crown chakra (the top of your head) as its powers are strongest there.

1 Sit in a comfortable chair with a straight spine or, if you prefer, sit cross-legged on a mat on the floor. Hold your piece of amethyst quietly in your hands and ask it to take away all the negative debris of the day that is clinging to you both physically and spiritually.
2 Sit quietly and let the crystal do its work for 10 minutes, then place it on your Third eye chakra to boost your intuitive powers. Finally, place it briefly on your Crown chakra to increase spiritual awareness.

AURA CLEANSING

If you did the Protecting your aura with colour exercise on page 42, you will have gained some protection from the upsets of the day. But for a calm evening, mist your aura (your spiritual energy field) with oils to clear away the daily irritations. If you leave your aura with any 'damage', your energy field becomes depleted and you will feel washed out. If this damage is not corrected, you become more vulnerable to illness. You may have also encountered an 'energy vampire' (see pages 21) during the day, who has drained precious energy from you. Make this cleansing routine a nightly ritual for your health and wellbeing.

AURA TIP
You can also cleanse your aura with a smouldering sage smudge stick (see pages 122–123).

CLEARING YOUR AURA

Spend a few minutes in a quiet space, such as your bedroom, to do this energetic cleansing.

1 Fill a large mister bottle (ideally glass) with water and mix in 5-6 drops of your oil.
2 Hold the bottle for a moment and ask for help to remove any negative vibrations from your aura. Then, stand upright and mist all around your body. Start at the top of your head, spraying down your left side to your feet. Spray down your right side, then down your front and send some to your back.
3 Rest briefly; then breathe in the fragrance of the oil and let it do its work.

OILS TO USE
Juniper and rosemary are powerful and invigorating cleansers.

Soothing lavender has the ability to bring your energy levels back to normal.

NIGHT VISUALIZATION

Once you have mastered the art of visualization
(see also page 82) you can use it in many ways to
create positive thoughts or images in your psyche.

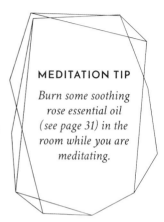

With this late-night exercise you can symbolically
dispose of any worries from the day in a beautiful
garden environment, so that your subconscious
mind is convinced they are really gone. When you
come to, you will have a lighter heart, a memory
of an idyllic place and you'll be able to go to sleep
soundly without a care in the world. You can also
use this technique to release a past hurt.

MEDITATION TIP

*Burn some soothing
rose essential oil
(see page 31) in the
room while you are
meditating.*

RETREATING TO A SPECIAL PLACE

Spend about 5-10 minutes nightly going to this special place to offload
your worries. Either hold or place in your pocket a rose quartz crystal
that you offer symbolically at the end of your visit.

1   Sit comfortably in a chair in a warm place. Close your eyes and
    breathe deeply. Visualize a beautiful summer garden. See the
    lush green lawns, the neat flower borders full of roses, carnations,
    chrysanthemums and other blooms. Smell the scented air and watch
    the flitting butterflies.
2   As you look around, you notice an empty flower border. Dig a small
    hole here with a nearby trowel. Now, visualize all your worries as a
    small black box. Place this box in the hole, covering it with soil.
3   Ask Mother Earth to accept your worries and transform them into
    joy. Leave her a gift of your rose quartz crystal and walk away
    feeling completely free. Slowly come to and open your eyes.

A CLEARING MEDITATION

Meditating shortly before you go to bed can calm an overactive mind and allow the brain to shut down properly in preparation for restorative sleep.

When you meditate (see also page 41) your brain activity slows down to the alpha wave level, which induces relaxation and brings healing. It is also a very cleansing process as it allows the subconscious mind to bring to the surface any suppressed information or feelings. If negative thoughts appear, maybe filling you with anger or pain, allow them to pass through you while breathing deeply; don't resist them, let them release through you.

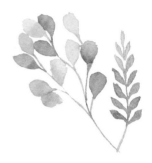

A NIGHT-TIME MEDITATION

Spend 5-10 minutes meditating each night to slow down your mind and to connect with your inner self.

1   Sit comfortably on an upright chair or cross-legged on a mat on the floor in a warm, dimly lit room. Start breathing deeply from your diaphragm to calm you.

2   Follow the meditation technique on page 41 and feel your mind and body relaxing as all your stresses leave your body. As thoughts or current concerns come to mind just let them float by, knowing that you will resolve any problems.

3   Acknowledge any inner or past emotions that surface, even if you want to resist them, as these deep-rooted hurts need healing and processing so that you can move on. After about 10 minutes, slowly open your eyes, feeling ready for a good night's sleep.

PURIFYING INCENSE

Burning scented incense in the late evening can relax you before going to bed. It can also enhance your mood, especially when combined with a night-time meditation (see page 133).

Incense has its roots with primitive humans, who found that certain burning woods released a pleasant aroma that affected the emotions (see also page 29). In the past, incense was used in many forms: as raw woods, crushed herbs, powders, pastes and even oils. The popular modern form, however, that will purify your living areas is incense sticks and cones; these are usually made from a mixture of fragrant plant oils, tree resins or gums, wood powders, herbs and spices.

TYPES OF INCENSE

There are combustible and non-combustible forms of incense.

The combustible forms – sticks, cones or coils – are the ones mainly used in the home. They contain saltpetre (potassium nitrate), which keeps the incense alight once lit.

Non-combustible incense will not burn by itself so needs to be placed on a combustible source. Incense suppliers sell charcoal blocks containing saltpetre specifically for burning this incense.

BURNING FRAGRANT INCENSE

Incense is not a strong cleanser for heavy energies but it enlivens and balances the ambience of a room to improve your mood.

1 Use a combustible incense fragrance (see right). Place your incense stick or cone firmly in or on its holder.
2 Light the tip. When it is burning well, blow out the flame so that the scented smoke wafts around the room. Sit nearby for a while and let the herbal aroma inspire your senses.

INCENSE TO USE

Jasmine or myrrh calm and prepare the body for sleep.

Cloves lift your emotions.

Vanilla energizes your body but soothes moods.

CALMING MANTRA

Performing a mantra in the late evening can help to clear your mind of the clutter and negative vibrations of the day and release any stress that you are still holding in your body. Chanting a chosen phrase continuously brings your body and mind into harmony (see page 52). The powerful vibration that the mantra creates corresponds to a specific spiritual energy and a state of consciousness. In time (this varies from person to person), the mantra absorbs and stills all other vibrations until your energy becomes totally in tune with the spiritual state represented by, and contained within, the mantra. Practising a mantra regularly can make you more in tune with yourself.

CHANTING A CHOSEN PHRASE CONTINUOUSLY BRINGS YOUR BODY AND MIND INTO HARMONY.

MANTRA FOR THE LATE EVENING

Chant this mantra regularly at night to get in touch with your spiritual self.

1 Sit cross-legged with a straight spine and relax your muscles (see page 41). Set any intent to cleanse your worries of the day or to help a current aim in your life.

2 Use the chant 'Om shrim mahalakshmiyei swaha' (approximate translation: salutations to that feminine energy which bestows all manner of wealth, and for which shrim is the seed). You can also abbreviate the chant to 'shrim', a word that basically means abundance (the more you say it the more abundance you will attract into your life).

3 Close your eyes and chant your phrase in a steady rhythm as you feel yourself relax. Chant for about 10 minutes, then slowly open your eyes and come to, feeling very at peace with yourself.

CLEARING ENERGIES

Your bedroom is a very important space. It is where you are very vulnerable as you rest your spirit for seven to eight hours a night, so the room's atmosphere needs to embrace you and make you feel very secure.

If the ambience is not right, you have been ill, had a disagreement with your partner in bed or if you have cleared out old clutter stored under the bed, the energy (*chi*) in your bedroom will be sticky and stagnant and may be affecting your sleep. Burning a soothing essential oil combination (see page 31) in your bedroom before sleep will clear the negativity in the air and leave a sensuous scent to encourage a deep and sound sleep.

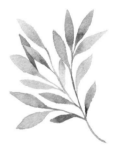

SPACE CLEARING THE BEDROOM

Burn your chosen essential oils for a short time in your bedroom before you sleep to calm your mind and spirit.

1   Place your oil mix in the bowl of a vaporizer and fill with water; vaporizers are often ceramic and are heated by a lit tea candle underneath the bowl. Alternatively, use an electric burner (see page 56).

2   Leave the oils burning for 10–15 minutes before you go to bed. Breathe in the delicious fragrance as you turn off or blow out the vaporizer's candle and slip into bed.

OIL COMBINATIONS TO USE

4 drops lavender oil, 2 drops geranium oil, 2 drops patchouli oil to calm, balance and inspire.

4 drops jasmine oil, 2 drops sandalwood oil, 2 drops ylang ylang to reduce stress and to soothe.

CLEANSING WORRIES

It is important to let go of any final niggling worries that are still circulating in your head before going to bed so that your mind slows down and clears, allowing rejuvenating sleep to come naturally.

Water is a wonderful cleanser and healer (see pages 72–73) that can be used in a waterfall visualization technique to purify and remove all the mental, psychic and physical disturbances that you still carry at the end of the day. The more you immerse yourself in the technique, seeing, feeling and tasting the water, the more effective it is.

CLEANSING TIP

For extra chakra cleansing, see the water changing to their seven colours as it flows down you (see page 49).

WATERFALL CLEANSER

Practise this technique for 5-10 minutes nightly to disperse any impurities that still cling to you.

1   Stand upright with a straight spine and relaxed shoulders. Close your eyes and see yourself standing beneath a running waterfall with crystal-clear water.
2   Feel the water raining down on your head; taste it as it passes your lips and then flows down your shoulders, over your stomach and down your legs. Sense any physical aches or pains disappearing with the flowing water.
3   Visualize your concerns and any energetic negativity being washed away with the healing water. See the water pooling at your feet and disappearing into the ground to be purified by Mother Earth. Slowly open your eyes and come to.

SALT PROTECTION

Salt has amazing purifying properties and since ancient times has been used in ceremonies to cleanse negativity. The large amount of salt used by the early Christians was thought to copy the Romans who liberally sprinkled it to repel evil demons or an unpleasant atmosphere. Its power lies partly in its antiseptic qualities and also in its crystalline structure, which is believed to realign the energy flowing through our bodies and our homes.

If you are experiencing bad dreams, having a difficult time at work or suffering emotional problems that are affecting your quality of sleep, you can use salt in the bedroom to offset these negative influences.

Keeping a bowl of salt by the bed or making a protective circle in the bedroom can make you secure and help you to sleep restfully.

SALT HAS AMAZING PURIFYING PROPERTIES AND SINCE ANCIENT TIMES HAS BEEN USED IN CEREMONIES TO CLEANSE NEGATIVITY.

PROTECTIVE SALT CIRCLES

A salt circle is an effective protective barrier when you are sleeping; this is the time when you are at your most vulnerable and open to suggestion. The circle will keep out other people's thoughts and feelings. It will also allow your mind to clear out any upsets or irritations that have occurred, so that you can process the events of the day in a healing and balanced way, leaving you to wake refreshed and energized.

PERFORM A SALT CEREMONY

Using salt in the bedroom can improve troubled sleep and dispel any lingering stagnant energies.

1 Take a handful of salt and hold it in your hand for a few seconds asking for help from the universe to improve how you sleep, resolve your troubles and protect you from any negativity.

2 Now, walk round your bed, sprinkling the salt in a large circle to enclose it. If you don't want to make a large circle, place some salt in a bowl next to your bed.

3 Throw away the salt every morning to remove all the impurities of the night and the previous day.

TYPES OF SALT TO USE

Unrefined sea salt (which evokes the power of the sea) and rock salt (which calls upon the power of the earth) are the best types to use for protection or purifying. Keep the salt in a sealed container until you want to use it, because as soon as it is exposed to the atmosphere it will start to absorb any impurities.

POSITIVE DREAMWORK

In the same way as you use visualization techniques (see pages 45 and 132) to embed positive thoughts in your subconscious mind or to produce a positive outcome to different dilemmas, you can use your dreams to find solutions to troublesome problems. Our dreams are often very graphic, detailed and emotional in their content as they relay messages to us from our subconscious. However, dreams use metaphorical symbols that you need to interpret and apply to your current situation.

YOU CAN USE YOUR DREAMS TO FIND SOLUTIONS TO TROUBLESOME PROBLEMS.

By holding your dilemma in your mind as you fall asleep, you leave your subconscious mind free to work on the problem and offer a solution in your dreams. In the morning, write down your dream and analyse its meaning.

DREAM SYMBOLS

If you receive symbols in a problem-solving dream that you do not understand, look them up in a dream book. Here are some common ones and their interpretation:

Fire can signal new beginnings, or if out of control the need to control ambition.

A hotel often signifies transition in a relationship.

Funerals can represent the end, or the need to end a phase of life.

A rainbow suggests good news or forgiveness.

Snow represents transformation; melting snow shows fears and obstacles disappearing.

Trains indicate you are receiving help on your journey.

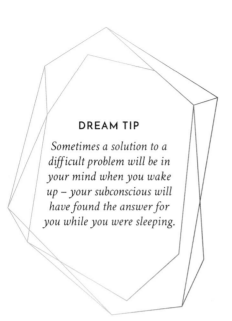

DREAM TIP

Sometimes a solution to a difficult problem will be in your mind when you wake up – your subconscious will have found the answer for you while you were sleeping.

DREAMING TO SOLVE PROBLEMS

Focus on the problem you want answered in your dreams for some minutes before going to sleep. Keep a pen and pad by your bed to write down your dream when you wake.

1   Sit up in bed, breathe deeply for a few minutes to relax you, then start to focus on the problem you want resolved. If it is a problem with your work, picture your desk or work environment, or if it is a relationship problem with your partner, lock on to his or her image.

2   Say what your problem is and what is worrying you about it. Ask for a clear-cut answer to your situation. Keep the imagery in your head as you fall asleep.

3   In the morning, write down the details of your dream in the first few minutes when you wake up as your brain loses the content very quickly. The answer may come in clear images or in symbols for you to interpret. Repeat the exercise for several nights if nothing is forthcoming on the first night.

INDEX

A
acupressure 12, 16
  early morning 53
  mid-morning 68-9
  pressure points 68
acupuncture 15, 64
aerobic exercise 8
affirmations see self-affirmations
alcohol 19
alternate nostril breathing 112-13
amethyst crystals 27, 32, 34, 35, 130
anger, letting go of 62-3
aquamarine crystals 32, 35, 83
aromatherapy see essential oils
aromatic showers 43
astra/emotional body 14
aura 13-14, 32
  clearing 131
  and colour therapy 48
  protecting 42
  spraying 117
aventurine crystals 61
Ayurvedic (Indian) medicine 10, 14

B
Bach flower remedies 28-29, 59
  stress and anger 64
barefoot walk on grass 74-5
bathing, candlelight 108-9
bedrooms, space clearing 136
blood-sugar levels 5, 6, 7, 26
books, sorting and storing 95
bosses, relationships with 22
breathing exercises 17, 26
  alternate nostril breathing 112-13
  breathing out stress 60-1
  centering 92
  cleansing breathing 80
  colour breathing energizer 49
  early morning 40
Bush flower remedies 28, 82
  emotional rebalancing 67
  stress and anger 64

C
caffeine 19-20
candlelight bathing 108-9
carbohydrates, and energy 7
centering 92
chakras 9, 14-15, 32
  and alternate nostril breathing 112

and anger 62
cleansing 137
and colour 14, 42, 48, 49, 98, 99
and crystals 32, 83, 91, 130
and head massage 101
chi 9, 53, 57, 116
  and drumming 118
  and water 73
chi kung/qigong 17, 78-9
child's pose 124-5
children 21
chromotherapy (colour therapy) 48
cigarette smoking 20
citrus oils 43
clapping 116
classes, dancing 115
cleansing breathing 80
clutter, clearing out 94-5
cobra posture 51
colleagues, relationships with 22
colour
  auras 13-14, 42
  chakras 14, 42, 48, 49, 98, 99
  dowsing for 99
  therapy 48-9, 98
computers, clearing 96
crystals 28, 34-5, 42
  anger remedies 64
  cleansing 34
  and computers 96
  dowsing for colour 99
  healing 83, 91, 130
  selecting 32
  and stress relief 61, 64
  and tree hugging 76
  uses and qualities 35

D
dancing 114-15
desk space, clearing 95
diet, and energy levels 8, 9, 19
Dog rose flower essence 29, 67
dowsing for colour 99
'draining' friendships 21
dreaming 140-1
drinks
  alcoholic 19
  caffeine-free 19-20
drumming 118-19

E
early morning 38-53
  absorbing colour energy 48-9

acupressure 53
aromatic showers 43
aura refreshment 42
breathing exercises 40
energy levels 39
fresh air 44
meditation 41
new day affirmation 47
tea 46
visualization 45
yoga 38, 50-1
earth energy 74-5
Eastern view of energy 6, 11-15
Elm Bach flower remedy 28, 59
emotional energy drains 20-2
energizer larder 27-25
  crystals 28, 32-5
  essential oils 28, 30-1
  flower remedies 28-9
  herbs and spices 32-3
  incense 29
  smudge sticks 29
energy blocks, removing 66
energy channels 5, 9, 10
energy levels 6, 8, 9
  early morning 39
  mid-morning 54
energy zappers 18-23
  emotional 20-2
  physical 18-20
  questionnaire 25, 36
  spiritual 23
energy-related therapies 16-17
essential oils 28, 30-1
  aura cleansing 131
  burners 56
  candlelight bathing 108-9
  hand massage 84
  mid-morning stress relief 55, 56-7
  neck and shoulder massage 110
  room purifying with 97, 117, 136
  stimulating 43
  stress and anger remedies 64
etheric body 14-15
evening refreshers 106-25
  breathing exercises 112-13
  candlelight bathing 108-9
  dancing 114-15
  neck and shoulder massage 110
  neck and shoulder stretching 111
  room purifying 116, 116-23
  yoga 124-5
exercises 10, 19

PICTURE CREDITS
Foliage watercolour illustrations:
  Teguh Kharyanda/Free Design
  Data

Geometric frames:
  Asmaa Rzq/Free Design
  Resources